Pain Control for Dental Practitioners

An Interactive Approach

DEMCO

Pain Control for Dental Practitioners

An Interactive Approach

Carlene Paarmann, RDH, MEd
Chair and Professor
Department of Dental Hygiene
Idaho State University

Royann Royer, RDH, MPH
Educator and Clinician
University of Alaska Anchorage
Alaska Native Medical Center

Wolters Kluwer | Lippincott Williams & Wilkins
Health
Philadelphia · Baltimore · New York · London
Buenos Aires · Hong Kong · Sydney · Tokyo

Executive Editor: John Goucher
Managing Editor: Kevin C. Dietz
Marketing Manager: Hilary Henderson
Associate Production Manager: Kevin P. Johnson
Design Coordinator: Stephen Druding
Cover Designer: Doris Bruey
Compositor: International Typesetting and Composition
Printer: Data Reproduction Corp.

Library of Congress Cataloging-in-Publication Data

Royer, Royann.
  Pain control for dental practitioners : an interactive approach / Royann Royer, Carlene Paarmann. — 1st ed.
      p. ; cm.
  Includes bibliographical references and index.
  ISBN-13: 978-0-7817-7914-2
  ISBN-10: 0-7817-7914-6
 1. Anesthesia in dentistry.   2. Local anesthesia.
3. Toothache—Treatment.   I. Paarmann, Carlene.   II. Title.
  [DNLM: 1. Dentistry—Programmed Instruction.   2. Facial Pain—therapy—Programmed Instruction.   3. Anesthetics—therapeutic use—Programmed Instruction.   WU 18.2 R897p 2007]
  RK510.R78 2007
  617.9'676—dc22

                                            2006036756

To purchase additional copies of this book call our customer service department at **(800) 638-3030** or fax orders to **(301) 824-7390**. International customers should call **(301) 714-2324**.

Visit Lippincott Williams & Wilkins on the Internet: http://www.lww.com. Lippincott Williams & Wilkins customer service representatives are available from 8:30 am to 6:00 pm, EST, Monday through Friday, for telephone access.

04 05
2 3 4 5 6 7 8 9 10

Preface

SCOPE/INTENT

Local anesthesia and nitrous oxide analgesia are essential to control pain in the everyday practice of dentistry and dental hygiene. These two pain control procedures involve skills that are being performed by more and more dental hygienists every year, as evidenced by the increasing number of states that now legally include the procedures in the scope of dental hygiene practice. Clinicians are seeking initial or refresher courses as new pharmacologic agents and technological advances and treatment of patients with medically compromising conditions affect pain control modalities in practice. As the demand for local anesthesia training has increased, so has the demand for faculty development, continuing education, teaching/learning materials, and readily accessible formal coursework.

   Having taught pain control procedures for many years, the authors and contributors of this teaching and learning package formulated the opinion that the available texts, while excellent, lacked certain information that contributes to the administration of safe and comfortable injections. For example, those textbooks might not contain content specific to the management of patient fear and anxiety, communication skills, risk management, or legal documentation as they relate to the administration of local anesthesia. Further, those reputable textbooks focus on either local anesthesia or nitrous oxide analgesia in the dental office. Because these two modalities often are used in conjunction with one another for pain control in the dental operatory, it is logical to include information on both procedures in one instructional package. Seemingly then, the old adage "necessity is the mother of invention" can be applied to explain the inspiration for a comprehensive training resource formatted as an instructional package.

INSTRUCTIONAL PACKAGE FORMAT AND FEATURES

The instructional package includes a CD-ROM and *Supplementary Clinical Manual*. Content is divided into five major sections. Each major section is further divided into "subsections," or "sections," as outlined:

Outline

   I. Local Anesthetic Agents (Carlene Paarmann and Royann Royer)
   1. Pain; Nerve Conduction
   2. Types and Action of Local Anesthetic Agents
   3. Pharmacology of Local Anesthetics
   4. Pharmacology of Vasoconstrictors
   5. Selection of Local Anesthetic Agents
   II. Injections (Carlene Paarmann and Royann Royer)
   1. Trigeminal Nerve/Anatomy of Significance
   2. Armamentarium
   3. Technique
   4. Selection of Injections
   5. Alternative Materials, Devices, and Techniques
   III. Potential Complications (Anita Herzog, Carlene Paarmann, and Royann Royer)
   1. Physical Evaluation (Health History Evaluation)
   2. Potential Complications

Within each section, course objectives, information on the CD, Predict Questions and Answers, and Quizzes (with Answer Key) have been compiled. Videoclips demonstrating the administration of individual local anesthesia injections and nitrous oxide technique supplement didactic instruction. The videoclips facilitate teaching and learning by eliminating the need to use live models for demonstration, thus making it possible for dental or dental hygiene students and practitioners to observe exactly how to administer local anesthesia without actually being in the clinical setting.

Assorted handouts, sample self-assessment and evaluation forms, and learning activities are also provided in the *Supplementary Clinical Manual*. The Learning Activities are designed to enhance instruction, retention, and use of information. Activities for each of the five major sections are presented in various forms (for example, simulations/patient scenarios, critiques, worksheets, evidence-based assignments).

These educational materials contribute to needs identified by dental and dental hygiene educators and serve as a prerequisite to clinical training required to achieve competence in these procedures. The instructional package is designed to fulfill coursework required for licensure in individual states or can serve as a review for either students or practitioners. This computer-based program is also valuable for busy practitioners who want to refresh their knowledge base quickly.

SUGGESTED USE OF THIS INSTRUCTIONAL PACKAGE

The following plan is suggested to gain maximum value from this package of information. Review the course objectives for the first section; read and study the corresponding information on the CD-ROM; answer the predict questions throughout the section; complete the quiz at the end of the section on the CD. An answer key provides immediate feedback for you to assess your comprehension of the material covered in that section. Review the objectives again and identify any unclear background/foundational information. Once clear, complete the learning activities associated with each section that are provided in the *Supplementary Clinical Manual*. Continue with this same process for each of the subsequent sections.

The *Supplementary Clinical Manual,* organized according to the corresponding section on the CD, is a valuable component of this instructional package. The manual provides charts or tables for a synopsis and quick review of the most pertinent material presented on the CD. This format serves as a quick reference guide for use in the clinical setting after completing this course. As mentioned previously, learning activities also are included in the manual to increase understanding of the information and enhance the reader's application of knowledge to practice. Many practitioners have laminated specific pages to have available for use as a chair-side reference. The manual also can be valuable when studying for quizzes and exams for each section or as a comprehensive review of all sections. Because several of the charts in the manual are best viewed in color and on one page they are also included in downloadable format in the CD ROM that accompany this *Supplementary Clinical Manual*.

Acknowledgments

There are so many people that have had an influence on or contributed to the development and completion of this project in a myriad of ways. Too many to list individually, the authors wish to collectively recognize and thank all of those individuals who helped us along the way. However, there are several people who deserve special recognition for their dedication to this project: Anita Herzog, RDH, MEd, Professor and Carole Christie, MCounsel, Associate Professor, Idaho State University, and J. Bryson McBratney DDS, University of Alaska Anchorage, for their expertise and contributions to the written materials in Sections III, IV, and V; Gretchen Hess (posthumously) and Susan Luthege for serving as patients/models during the filming of injection videos; Marty Welch for filming and editing the videos; Laura Brewer and the many people at the Instructional Technology Resource Centers at both Idaho State University and the University of Alaska Anchorage. We also want to recognize our many students over the years—both undergraduate and continuing education participants—who have shared their comments and constructive criticism of the written materials, charts, and videoclips. We are indebted to all of you. It is our sincere desire that the information contained in this packet benefits today's students and practitioners as well as many future clinicians. We welcome suggestions and comments that might improve future editions.

Carlene Paarman RDH, MEd and Royann Royer RDH, MPH

I would like to express my sincere gratitude to my husband Tom and daughter Michala for their support and encouragement throughout the many years this project has taken to come to fruition. I would like to thank my many friends and colleagues at the University of Alaska and Southcentral Foundation who not only gave me support, they often reviewed and/or participated in the development process of this long-term project. I could not have done it without you! I would also like to recognize a very special individual, JJ Kovaleski, who is no longer with us and would have been very proud to see this project completed.

Royann Royer RDH, MPH

To my family, friends, and extraordinary colleagues at Idaho State University, I extend my sincere appreciation for the support and encouragement you offered throughout this seemingly endless project. A special thank you is extended to my mother who lovingly and singlehandedly raised her children and taught them the value of hard work and patience. Without those attributes, this project could not have been completed!

Carlene Paarman RDH, MEd

Table of Contents

Key to Quizzes/Self Tests

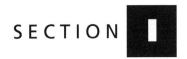

Local Anesthetic Agents

Summary of Factors Affecting Pain Reaction Thresholds

One, several, or all of the following factors have an impact on an individual's pain reaction threshold. Descriptions provided are **generalizations**.

CHARACTERISTIC	IMPORTANCE
Emotional state	Patients who are more emotionally insecure generally have lower pain reaction thresholds than patients who are not experiencing emotional "lows."
Fatigue	Patients who are well rested and who have had a good night's sleep previous to an unpleasant experience will have a much higher pain reaction threshold than individuals who are tired.
Age	The older population tends to have a prevalence of fear and pain associated with dentistry lower than that of children.
Racial/nationality/ cultural characteristics	Most research studies indicate that culture, more than race, has a major influence on pain reaction. Individuals turn toward their social environment to determine what reactions are appropriate to convey; they receive validation from their cultural group—primarily from their family members.
Gender	Research studies generally report that men have a higher pain reaction threshold than women. It should be noted that any differences are not significant enough that one could predict the level of fear an individual might experience based solely on gender.
Fear and apprehension	The more fearful or apprehensive a patient, the lower the patient reaction threshold. These individuals frequently skip their appointments altogether, compromising their dental health.

Source: Compiled from Bennet (1984), Bouffard (1999), Gadbury-Amyot (2000), Milgrom et al. (1995)

Summary of Common Local Anesthetic Agents and Vasoconstrictors

The information contained in the following table was compiled primarily from Malamed's *Handbook of Local Anesthesia* (2004), Moore (1990), and manufacturer's package inserts (1990, 1993, 2000, 2003)

GENERIC NAME	LIDOCAINE			MEPIVACAINE		PRILOCAINE		ARTICAINE		BUPIVA-CAINE
Common trade name(s)	Lidocaine HCl Xylocaine HCl	Lidocaine HCl Xylocaine HCl	Lidocaine HCl Xylocaine HCl	Carbocaine Polocaine	Carbocaine Polocaine	Citanest Plain	Citanest Forte	Septocaine/ Zorcaine	Septocaine	Marcaine
Concentration of anesthetic agent (%)	2%	2%	2%	3%	2%	4%	4%	4%	4%	0.5%
Amount of anesthetic agent (mg/mL)	20 mg/mL	20 mg/mL	20 mg/mL	30 mg/mL	20 mg/mL	40 mg/mL	40 mg/mL	40 mg/mL	40 mg/mL	5 mg/mL
Amount of anesthetic agent per carpule (mg/cartridge)	36 mg	36 mg	36 mg	54 mg	36 mg	72 mg	72 mg	68 mg (1.7 mL cartridges)	68 mg (1.7 mL cartridges)	9 mg
Maximum dose of anesthetic agent (mg/lb body weight)	2 mg/lb	2 mg/lb	2 mg/lb	2 mg/lb	2 mg/lb	2.7 mg/lb	2.7 mg/lb	3.2 mg/lb	3.2 mg/lb	0.6 mg/lb
Maximum recommended dose (MRD) anesthetic per appointment	300 mg	300 mg	300 mg	300 mg	300 mg	400 mg	400 mg	500 mg	500 mg	90 mg
Vasoconstrictor	—	Epinephrine	Epinephrine	—	Levonordefrin (Neocobefrin)	—	Epinephrine	Epinephrine	Epinephrine	Epinephrine
Concentration of vasoconstrictor	—	1:50,000	1:100,000	—	1:20,000	—	1:200,000	1:100,000	1:200,000	1:200,000
Concentration of vasoconstrictor (mg/mL)	—	0.02 mg/mL	0.01 mg/mL	—	0.05 mg/mL	—	0.005 mg/mL	0.01 mg/mL	0.005 mg/mL	0.005 mg/mL
Amount of vasoconstrictor per cartridge (mg)	—	0.036 mg	0.018 mg	—	0.09 mg	—	0.009 mg	0.017 mg (1.7 mL cartridges)	0.008 mg	0.009 mg
Maximum recommended dose vasoconstrictor (MRD) per appointment	—	0.2 mg	0.2 mg	—	1.0 mg	—	0.2 mg	0.2 mg	0.2 mg	0.2 mg

(continued)

GENERIC NAME	LIDOCAINE			MEPIVACAINE		PRILOCAINE		ARTICAINE		BUPIVA-CAINE
Agent limiting max. volume for healthy patient	Lidocaine	Epinephrine	Lidocaine	Mepivacaine	Mepivacaine	Prilocaine	Prilocaine	Articaine	Articaine	Bupivacaine
Number of cartridges needed to reach MRD of limiting agent (healthy patient)	8.3	5.5	8.3	5.5	8.3	5.5	5.5	7.3	7.3	10
pKa	7.9	7.9	7.9	7.6	7.6	4.9	7.9			8.1
Color coding: band on cylinder (as of 6/2003)	Light blue	Green	Red	Tan	Brown	Black	Yellow	Gold	Silver	Blue
Duration	Short	Inter-mediate	Inter-mediate	Short	Inter-mediate	Short	Inter-mediate	Inter-mediate	Inter-mediate	Long
Pulpal tissues	5–10 min	60 min	60 min	20–40 min	60–90 min	Infil-tration: 5–10 min Block: 40–60 min	60–90 min	Infil-tration: 60 min Block: 120 min	Infil-tration: 60 min Block: 120 min	1.5–5 h
Soft tissues	1–2 h	3–5 h	3–5 h	2–3 h	3–5 h	Infil-tration: 1.5–2 h Block: 2–4 h	3–8 h	3–6 h	3–6 h	4–9 h
Agent limiting max volume for vasoconstrictor-sensitive patient	Lidocaine	Epinephrine	Epinephrine	Mepivacaine	Levonordefrin	Prilocaine	Epinephrine	Epinephrine	Epinephrine	Epinephrine
Number of cartridges needed to reach MRD of limiting agent (vasoconstrictor-sensitive patient)	8.3	1.1	2.2	5.5	2.2	5.5	4.4	2.35	4.4	4.4

Note: Articaine 4% is packaged in a 1.7 ml. cartridge; therefore, 40 × 1.7 = 68 mg. articaine/cartridge and .01 × 1.7 = .017 mg epinephrine 1:100:000 OR .005 × 1.7 = .0085 mg. 1:200,000/cartridge

Milligrams of LA in Dental Cartridge
0.5% = 5 mg/mL × 1.8 = 9 mg/cartridge
2% = 20 mg/mL × 1.8 = 36 mg/cartridge
3% = 30 mg/mL × 1.8 = 54 mg/cartridge
4% = 40 mg/mL × 1.8 = 72 mg/cartridge

Milligrams of Vasoconstrictor in Dental Cartridge
1:20,000 .05 mg/mL × 1.8 = .09 mg/cartridge
1:50,000 .02 mg/mL × 1.8 = .036 mg/cartridge
1:100,000 .01 mg/mL × 1.8 = .018 mg/cartridge
1:200,000 .005 mg/mL × 1.8 = .009 mg/cartridge

Maximum Dosage of Vasoconstrictors		
	HEALTHY ADULT	**MEDICALLY COMPROMISED**
epinephrine	.2 mg/appoint.	.04 mg/appoint
1:50,000	5.5 cartridges	1 cartridge
1:100,000	11 cartridges	2 cartridges
1:200,000	22 cartridges	4 cartridges
levonordephrin	1 mg/appoint.	.2 mg/appoint
1:20,000	11 cartridges	2.2 cartridges

Summary of Common Topical Anesthetics*

TYPE	BRAND NAME EXAMPLES	FORM	CONCENTRATION	ONSET/DURATION
Esters	Benzocaine	Gel	20%	1–2 min/5–15 min
		Liquid	20%	30 s/10–20 min
		Patch	18%	<2min/20 min
	Cetacaine	Spray	2% tetracaine 14% benzocaine	30 s/30–60 min
	Freeze	Spray	15% tetracaine 18% benzocaine	30 s/60 min
Amides	Lidocaine	Ointment	5%	1–2 min/5–15 min
	Lidocaine Dentipatch	Patch	10–20%	5 min/30–45 min
EMLA (eutectic mixture of 2.5% lidocaine and 2.5% prilocaine)	EMLA	Cream (not FDA approved for oral mucosa)	2.5% lidocaine; 2.5% prilocaine	5 min/15–20 min
	Oraquix	Liquid that turns to gel at body temp.	2.5% lidocaine; 2.5% prilocaine	30 s/20–30 min
Dyclonine	Not available except through apothecary pharmacy	Liquid	0.5%	2 min/30–60 min

*Information compiled from package inserts and *ADA Guide to Dental Therapeutics,* 4th ed. For complete information (dosage, side effects, etc), see CD Section I.2.

Summary of Toxic Reactions: Signs, Symptoms, and Management

REACTIONS TO ELEVATED LEVELS OF LOCAL ANESTHESIA

TYPE	SIGNS	SYMPTOMS
Minimal → moderate blood levels of anesthetic	**CNS:** Stimulation Excitedness Apprehension Talkativeness Confusion Nervousness Slurred, stuttered speech Muscular twitching and tremor **CVS:** Elevated blood pressure, heart rate, respiratory rate	Lightheadedness Restlessness Nervousness Dizziness Headache Blurred vision Tinnitus Oral parasthesia Chills/flushing Drowsiness Disorientation
High blood levels of anesthetic	**CNS:** Generalized tonic-clonic seizures Generalized CNS depression **CVS:** Fallen blood pressure, heart rate, respiratory rate	Loss of consciousness

REACTIONS TO ELEVATED LEVELS OF VASOCONSTRICTORS

TYPE	SIGNS	SYMPTOMS
Vasocon-strictor overdose reaction	Pallor Diaporesis Dyspnea Tremor Sharp rise in systolic blood pressure Elevated heart rate Possible cardiac dysrhyth-mias	Nervousness Tremor Fear Perspiration Anxiety Dizziness Restlessness Throbbing headache Weakness Respiratory difficulty

Source: Compiled from Malamed (2004), Yagiela (1999), Hass (2002), and Finder (2002)

Management of Local Anesthetic Overdose

Management of Vasoconstrictor Overdose

Terminate dental treatment	Terminate dental treatment
Position patient supine	Position patient upright
Maintain airway and provide supplemental oxygen	Maintain airway and provide supplemental oxygen (*exception:* hyperventilation)
Summon EMS	Reassure patient
Protect patient who is seizing from injury without restraining	Monitor vital signs
Monitor vital signs	Summon EMS if symptoms persist for more than 5 min
Provide basic life support	Continue to provide basic life support while awaiting EMS

Even if a patient is not having difficulty breathing, oxygen relieves symptoms and improves blood oxygen levels and perfusion. This can prevent loss of consciousness.

Adapted from Biron CR, *Adverse Reactions to Local Anesthetics,* RDH October 2000.

SECTION I LEARNING ACTIVITIES

PAIN REACTION THRESHOLD OBSERVATIONS

1. Identify pain thresholds and determine reasons for their particular level of pain on five of your patients tomorrow (both high and low pain reaction thresholds).

Patient 1 _____

Patient 2 _____

Patient 3 _____

Patient 4 _____

Patient 5 _____

LOCAL ANESTHETIC PRACTICE CALCULATIONS

DIRECTIONS: Be sure to show all calculations. A key is provided for you to check your responses after completing this practice activity. Answers are based on the MRD's listed on the "Summary of Common Local Anesthetic Agents and Vasoconstrictors" chart found in this manual on page 2 and 3.

1. a. How many milligrams of Xylocaine 2% can be administered to a 120-lb patient?

_____

   b. How many carpules would be administered?

_____

2. You have administered 3.5 carpules of Carbocaine 3% to your patient. How many milligrams have you administered?

_____

3. a. How many milligrams of anesthetic are contained in 5 carpules of Citanest Forte?

_____

   b. How many milligrams of vasoconstrictor? Name the vasoconstrictor.

_____

4. What is the maximum number of carpules of lidocaine you can use if you have already given 2 cartridges of 3% mepivacaine to a 120-lb. healthy female?

_____

5. Calculate the MRD and number of cartridges you could administer safely during one appointment for:
   a. For a 185-lb healthy adult
   b. For a 90-lb 12-year-old healthy boy
   c. For a 130-lb healthy woman

DRUG AVAILABLE:	A. 185-LB HEALTHY ADULT		B. 90-LB 12-YR.-OLD BOY		C. 130-LB WOMAN	
	MRD	CARPULES	MRD	CARPULES	MRD	CARPULES
3% Mepivacaine						
2% Mepivacaine						
0.5% Bupivacaine						
4% Prilocaine						
4% Articaine						

SELECTION OF ANESTHETIC SCENARIOS

1. Select an appropriate anesthetic and provide rationale for your response to each of the following:
   a. What is an appropriate anesthetic to administer to a 75-lb healthy child who has a 60-min appointment to receive MOD (mesio-occluso-distal) on teeth A and B.

   b. Your patient requires extensive root planning at a 3-hour appointment. There are no medical history complications.

   c. Your 10:00 A.M. patient is appointed for an extraction of tooth #2. He has high blood pressure and is being evaluated by his physician for diabetes.

2. Research and evaluate five different types of topical anesthetics (spray, ointment, injectable, lollipop, patches). Would you recommend these products to a peer? Why or why not?

3. Evidence based decision making (EBDM): Discuss the controversy surrounding the use of articaine for mandibular block injections. Provide evidence for pros and cons of use.

ANSWER KEY TO CALCULATIONS

1. a. How many milligrams of xylocaine 2% can be administered to a 120 lb. patient?
      MRD: 120 lb $\times$ 2 mg/lb = **240 mg**
   b. How many carpules would be administered?
      240 mg $\div$ 36 mg = **6.6 cartridges**
2. You have administered 3.5 carpules of Carbocaine 3% to your patient. How many milligrams have you administered?
      54 mg $\times$ 3.5 = **189 mg**
3. a. How many milligrams of anesthetic are contained in 5 carpules of Citanest Forte?
      72 mg $\times$ 5 = **360 mg**
   b. How many milligrams of vasoconstrictor? Name the vasoconstrictor.
      0.009 $\times$ 5 = **.045 mg**   1:200,000 **epinephrine**

4. What is the maximum number of carpules of lidocaine you can use if you have already given 2 cartridges of 3% mepivicaine to a 120-lb healthy woman?

MRD = 120 × 2 = 204 mg
Already given 2 × 54 mg = 108 mg
Can give 204 − 108 = 132 mg additional
132 mg. ÷ 36 mg/cartridge = **3.66 cartridges**

5. Calculate the MRD and number of cartridges you could administer safely during one appointment for:
a. For a 185-lb healthy adult
b. For a 90-lb 12-year-old healthy boy
c. For a 130-lb healthy woman

DRUG AVAILABLE:	A. 185-LB HEALTHY ADULT		B. 90-LB 12-YR.-OLD BOY		C. 130-LB WOMAN	
	MRD	CARPULES	MRD	CARPULES	MRD	CARPULES
3% Mepivacaine	300 mg	5.5	180 mg	3.3	260 mg	4.8
2% Mepivacaine	300 mg	8.3	180 mg	5	260 mg	7.2
.5% Bupivacaine	90 mg	10	54 mg	6	78 mg	8.6
4% Prilocaine	400 mg	5.5	243 mg	3.4	351 mg	4.8
4% Articaine	500 mg	7.3	288 mg	4.2	416 mg	6.1

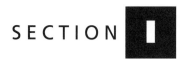

Local Anesthetic Agents/Quizzes

Pain/Nerve Conduction

1. In the depolarized nerve cell, there are more positively charged ions outside the cell than inside because the nerve membrane is relatively impermeable to sodium.
   a. True
   b. False

2. The minimal threshold stimulus required to excite a C-fiber will also be sufficient to stimulate an A-fiber.
   a. True
   b. False

3. The physioanatomical process that transmits pain from the free nerve endings to the central nervous system (CNS) is:
   a. Psychogenic pain reaction
   b. Pain reaction threshold
   c. Pain reaction
   d. Pain perception

4. When energy for conduction is derived from the nerve cell membrane itself and is no longer dependent on the stimulus for continuance, the conduction is considered to be:
   a. Below the minimal threshold level
   b. Above the minimal threshold level
   c. Self-propagating
   d. In the absolute refractory period

5. The relative refractory period occurs during the fraction of a millisecond when a nerve fiber can be excited only by a much stronger stimulus than the initial stimulus.
   a. True
   b. False

6. Nerve fibers are divided according to size and conduction velocity or speed. The two fibers we are concerned with in dentistry are:
   a. A-alpha and C
   b. A-alpha and A-delta
   c. A-delta and C
   d. A-delta and B

7. Nerve conduction along a myelinated nerve expends more energy due to increased speed and intensity.
   a. True
   b. False

8. The absolute refractory period occurs during the fraction of a millisecond when a nerve fiber can be exited only by a much stronger stimulus than the initial stimulus.
   a. True
   b. False

9. The larger the diameter the nerve fiber, the more likely that fiber is to be myelinated.
   a. True
   b. False

10. Saltatory conduction refers to:
    a. Rapid transmission of nerve impulses along a myelinated nerve fiber
    b. Diffusion of sodium chloride into the nerve cell during impulse conduction
    c. Conduction of an impulse along a nonmyelinated nerve at the nodes of Ranvier
    d. None of the above

11. A group of nerve fibers bundled together is referred to as:
    a. Nerve trunk
    b. A ganglion
    c. Nociceptors
    d. Paraperiosteal nerves

12. A group of cell bodies (nerve) bundled together are referred to as:
    a. A nerve trunk
    b. Nociceptors
    c. Ruffini end organs
    d. Pacini corpuscles
    e. A ganglion

13. Assume for a moment that all nerve fibers affected in an area are the same size (e.g., A-delta). The difference in pain intensity is derived from:
    a. The number of individual cells excited
    b. The frequency of excitation (duration of stimulus)
    c. The strength of the stimulus
    d. a and b
    e. All of the above

14. When a stimulus of sufficient intensity to create an impulse is applied to a nerve ending, the permeability of the cell membrane is altered and depolarization is initiated. Which of the following does *not* happen *during* depolarization?
    a. Sodium rapidly passes through the nerve cell membrane into the axoplasm
    b. Sodium is pumped out of the nerve cell by the sodium pump
    c. Nerve transmembrane potential is decreased to initiate an action potential
    d. a and c

15. In myelinated nerves, local anesthetics must diffuse through the myelin sheath to reach the nerve membrane to block the nerve impulse.
    a. True
    b. False

16. Saltatory conduction is a term that refers to:
    1. Impulse conduction which leaps from node to node
    2. Impulse conduction in a slow, creeping forward direction
    3. Impulse conduction in myelinated nerves
    4. Impulse conduction in unmyelinated nerves
    5. Impulse conduction with a hydrochloride salt

Answer Choices:
a. 1 and 4
b. 2 and 3
c. 1 and 3 —
d. 3 and 5
e. 4 and 5

17. When a nerve is at rest, which of the following statements is true?
    a. Na$^+$ concentration is highest inside the cell
    b. The cell membrane is more negative on the outside
    c. The cell membrane can be excited if a stimulus is intense enough to initiate an impulse ___
    d. Regardless of the stimulus intensity, the nerve cannot respond to a stimulus when in this particular state

18. Your first patient of the morning stayed up all night studying for his 1:00 history exam. He will most likely have a higher pain reaction threshold than usual.
    a. True
    b. False —

19. As you prepare to anesthetize him, your patient clenches his hands and beads of perspiration form on his upper lip and brow. He is exhibiting:
    a. Pain perception
    b. Pain reaction —
    c. Pain resistance
    d. Pain reflex
    e. Pain rebound

20. The administration of local anesthesia to control pain is an example of:
    a. Raising the pain reaction threshold
    b. Cortical depression
    c. Interrupting pain perception—
    d. Removing the cause of the pain
    e. Psychosomatic pain control

21. Juanita Rodriquez, from Guadalajara, will most likely have a higher pain reaction threshold than Sue Smith, who was raised in Fairbanks, Alaska.
    a. True
    b. False —

22. The most similarity of nerve membrane electrochemical potential exists between:
    a. Polarization and depolarization
    b. Depolarization and repolarization
    c. Polarization and repolarization —
    d. Polarization and the absolute refractory period

23. The resting potential of a nerve fiber is:
    a. Maintained in part by the sodium pump
    b. Maintained in part by the permeability of the cell membrane
    c. An electrochemical gradient of –70 to –90 mV
    d. All of the above —

24. Psychogenic pain may be most accurately described as:
    a. Dull pain which is limited to the area of origin
    b. Discomfort for which no organic cause can be determined —
    c. Diffuse in nature and difficult to localize
    d. Sharp, burning, intense localized pain

25. Referred pain may be expressed in some part of the body other than its physiological point of origin.
    a. True —
    b. False

Types and Action of Local Anesthetic Agents

1. Which of the following factors significantly improves the effectiveness of a local anesthetic agent?
   a. Protein-binding capability of local anesthetic agent
   b. Perineurium along the nerve fiber
   c. Lipid solubility of local anesthetic agent
   d. a and c
   e. All of the above —

2. What are the base molecules responsible for in local anesthetics?
   a. Diffusion of local anesthesia through the nerve membrane
   b. Onset time of local anesthesia
   c. Duration of local anesthesia
   d. a and b
   e. a and c

3. What are cation molecules responsible for in local anesthetics?
   a. Diffusion of local anesthesia through nerve membranes
   b. Binding at the receptor sites in the ion channels
   c. Reduction or prevention of sodium ions through the nerve membrane
   d. a and c
   e. b and c

4. Which of the following circumstances would cause the greatest decrease in pH and therefore reduce effectiveness of local anesthetic?
   a. Normal tissue using local anesthetic with epinephrine.
   b. Inflamed tissue using local anesthetic without epinephrine.
   c. Inflamed tissue using local anesthesia with epinephrine.
   d. Inflamed tissue using local anesthetic with levonordefrin.
   e. c and d

5. Mepivacaine has the lowest pKa of most local anesthetics. This would indicate which of the following?
   a. The local anesthetic has a high percentage of base molecules
   b. The local anesthetic has a high percentage of cations
   c. The onset of action would be slow
   d. The pH of the tissue will increase after the injection
   e. b and c

6. Which of the following anesthetic/anesthetics are available in the US with 1:200,000 epinephrine?
   a. Lidocaine
   b. Mepivacaine
   c. Prilocaine
   d. Bupivacaine
   e. c and d

7. Topical anesthetics are not manufactured in which of the following forms?
   a. Esters
   b. Amides
   c. Amides with vasoconstrictors
   d. Ketones
   e. c and d

8. Why are topical anesthetics manufactured in higher concentrations than local anesthetics?
   a. More base molecules are needed to allow the drug to diffuse through mucous membranes
   b. They cannot produce toxicity when applied topically
   c. Decreased amounts are applied topically than when injected locally
   d. They do not contain vasoconstrictors
   e. c and d

9. Which anesthetic has a pulpal anesthesia of 10 min for an infiltration injection and 60 min for a block injection?
   a. Lidocaine
   b. Mepivacaine plain
   c. Prilocaine plain
   d. Prilocaine with 1:200,000 epinephrine
   e. Mepivacaine with 1:20,000 neocobefrin

10. Match the following anesthetic drug (generic name) with the appropriate product (trade) name:

TRADE NAME	GENERIC NAME
_____Xylocaine	A. Lidocaine
_____Septocaine	B. Mepivacaine
_____Carbocaine	C. Prilocaine
_____Citanest	D. Bupivacaine
_____Marcaine	E. Articaine

11. Which of the following anesthetics has the shortest duration of action?
   a. Carbocaine 3%
   b. Carbocaine 2% 1: 20,000
   c. Marcaine 0.5% 1:200,000
   d. Xylocaine 2% 1:100,000
   e. Citanest 4% 1:200,000

Pharmacology of Local Anesthetics

SECTION 1-3

1. In a healthy individual, which system is the most sensitive to the actions of the local anesthetic agent?
   a. Cardiovascular
   b. Central nervous
   c. Respiratory
   d. Digestive
   e. Immune

2. Three cartridges of local anesthetic contain how many milliliters of solution?
   a. 3.6 mL
   b. 5.4 mL
   c. 6 mL
   d. 7.2 mL
   e. 8.5 mL

3. Where is the primary location for biotransformation or metabolism of amide-type anesthetics?
   a. Kidney
   b. Plasma
   c. Liver
   d. Adrenal cortex
   e. Lungs

4. What is the maximum safe/recommended dose (number of carpules) of Mepivacaine 3% for a normal healthy adult, weighing 160 lb or more?
   a. 4
   b. 5.5
   c. 6.5
   d. 7.5
   e. 8

5. Liver disease is a relative contraindication to which local anesthetic agent?
   a. Esters
   b. Amides
   c. Benzocaine
   d. a and b
   e. Liver disease would not affect utilization of local anesthetic agent

6. The type of local anesthesia and an individual's weight are important in determining potential toxicity. Which other factor may affect toxicity level?
   a. Age
   b. Intravascular injection
   c. Pathologic conditions/diseases patient may have
   d. a and c
   e. All of the above

7. Which injection technique is the *most* important in decreasing systemic absorption of local anesthetic?
   a. Injecting rapidly
   b. Injecting slowly
   c. Selecting a local anesthetic without epinephrine
   d. Depositing the solution intramuscularly
   e. Aspirating prior to reaching the target area of the injection

8. Local anesthetics without vasoconstrictors at toxic levels may produce cardiovascular symptoms which appear as:
   a. Decrease in blood pressure
   b. Increase in blood pressure
   c. Cardiac dysrhythmias
   d. Increased contraction force
   e. b and d

9. How many milligrams of lidocaine are in 1 mL of 2% lidocaine?
   a. 2 mg
   b. 18 mg
   c. 20 mg
   d. 1.8 mg
   e. 36 mg

10. Three carpules of 4% prilocaine anesthetic solution would contain how many milligrams of anesthetic agent?
    a. 30 mg
    b. 90 mg
    c. 120 mg
    d. 162 mg
    e. 216 mg

Pharmacology of Vasoconstrictors

SECTION 1-4

1. A vasoconstrictor that has a 1:100,000 concentration has how many milligrams per milliliter of vasoconstrictor in that solution?
   a. 0.001 mg/mL
   b. 0.05 mg/mL
   c. 0.01 mg/mL
   d. 1 mg/mL
   e. None of the above

2. Which of the following conditions would be a relative contraindication to the use of a vasoconstrictor?
   a. Patient with a history of a heart attack 3 years ago, no current complications
   b. Patient with hyperthyroid condition, on medication
   c. Patient taking a nonselective beta blocker heart medication
   d. b and c
   e. All of the above

3. Which of the following symptoms would distinguish if a patient is having a toxic response to the local anesthetic drug or the vasoconstrictor at moderate overdose levels?
   a. Headaches
   b. Tremors
   c. Blood pressure
   d. Breathing difficulty
   e. Loss of consciousness

4. According to most of the literature, levonordefrin at 1:20,000 concentration produces which of the following responses when compared to epinephrine at 1:100,000?
   a. Less cardiac response than epinephrine
   b. Less central nervous system (CNS) response than epinephrine
   c. Approximately the same cardiac and CNS response as epinephrine
   d. Significant increase in cardiac and CNS response than epinephrine
   e. a and b

5. The maximum number of carpules of anesthetic in a "normal, healthy" patient is usually restricted by what factor contained in the local anesthetic?
   a. Vasoconstrictor
   b. Local anesthetic drug
   c. Sodium bisulfites
   d. pH of the local anesthetic
   e. b and d

6. The maximum safe dose of the vasoconstrictor epinephrine, at one setting, is approximately 0.2 mg for the "normal" healthy adult patient. In a 1:100,000 solution, this would translate into how many carpules?
   a. 2 carpules
   b. 4 carpules
   c. 8 carpules
   d. 11 carpules
   e. 15 carpules

7. Which of the following vasoconstrictors is most likely to cause necrosis and sloughing of tissues?
   a. Epinephrine 1:50,000
   b. Epinephrine 1:100,000
   c. Epinephrine 1:200,000
   d. Levonodefrin 1:20,000
   e. a and d

8. Vasoconstrictors are effective for increasing duration of local anesthetics because:
   a. Of their primary action on beta receptors
   b. Of their primary action on alpha receptors
   c. The contraction of smooth muscles inside blood vessels
   d. Of their effect on pH of tissues
   e. b and c

9. If a local anesthetic with a 1:200,000 concentration of epinephrine is being utilized on a patient with heart disease, what would be the maximum safe dose?
   a. Approximately 1 carpule
   b. Approximately 2 carpules
   c. Approximately 4 carpules
   d. Approximately 8 carpules
   e. Approximately 11 carpules

10. How much epinephrine does 2% lidocaine with 1:100,000 epinephrine contain compared with the 1:50,000 solution of epinephrine?
    a. Twice
    b. Half
    c. One fourth
    d. One third
    e. None of the above

Selection of Local Anesthetic Agents

1. Which is a vasoconstrictor used in topical anesthetic solutions?
   a. Benzocaine
   b. Epinephrine
   c. Levonordefrin
   d. Lidocaine
   e. None of the above

2. Assuming 300 mg is the maximum recommended dose, how many carpules of Carbocaine 2% can be administered to a 175-lb, healthy man before reaching the maximum recommended dose (MRD)?
   a. 11.1 cartridges
   b. 10.1 cartridges
   c. 8.3 cartridges
   d. 6.6 cartridges
   e. 5.5 cartridges

3. Which of the following has the shortest duration of *pulpal* anesthesia when administering a block injection?
   a. Lidocaine plain
   b. Bupivacaine plain
   c. Prilocaine plain
   d. Mepivacaine 3%

4. Which of the following is the longest acting anesthetic solution?
   a. Lidocaine
   b. Prilocaine
   c. Mepivacaine
   d. Bupivacaine

5. Match the local anesthetic agent with the average pulpal or soft tissue length of duration.

   _____Lidocaine plain   A. 50–90 min pulpal, 3–5 h soft tissue

   _____Mepivacaine 2%   B. 90–180 min pulpal, 4–9 h soft tissue

   _____Mepivacaine 3%   C. 20 min pulpal, 2–3 h soft tissue

   _____Prilocaine plain   D. 5–10 min pulpal, 1–2 h soft tissue

   _____Bupivacaine   E. Block: 40–60 min pulpal, 2–4 h soft tissue

6. Which anesthetic is best for a patient requiring extensive root planing at one 3-hour appointment?
   a. Citanest plain
   b. 3% Carbocaine
   c. 2% Xylocaine 1:100,000
   d. Marcaine, 1:200,000

7. Jackie Jackson comes into the office for extraction of tooth 15. Medical history: 60 years old, overweight, apprehensive, blood pressure 160/94, pulse 89, respiration 22. Under treatment for high blood pressure and weight reduction. You call her physician who gives you permission to treat her with necessary precautions. You choose to administer prilocaine with vasoconstrictor. What drug is the limiting factor for anesthetizing this patient?
   a. Citanest
   b. Mepivacaine
   c. Epinephrine
   d. Levonordefrin

8. Five carpules of lidocaine 2%, 1:100,000 have been administered to the patient. This patient has a history of heart disease, so the MRD for epinephrine has been reduced to 0.04 mg. Has the MRD for the vasoconstrictor been exceeded?
   a. Yes
   b. No

9. Which anesthetic/anesthetics are available in the US with 1:200,000 epinephrine?
   a. Lidocaine
   b. Mepivacaine
   c. Prilocaine
   d. Articaine
   e. c and d

10. Due to its short duration, which anesthetic is clinically useless in most circumstances without the addition of a vasoconstrictor?
    a. Mepivacaine
    b. Lidocaine
    c. Prilocaine
    d. Articaine
    e. Bupivacaine

11. Which anesthetic has 1:200,000 epinephrine, a short half-life, moderate length of anesthesia, and rapid biotransformation?
    a. Lidocaine
    b. Articaine
    c. Mepivacaine
    d. Marcaine
    e. Bupivacaine

12. What preservative is included in lidocaine 2% plain (no vasoconstrictor) to prolong its shelf life?
    a. No preservative is included
    b. Sodium bisulfite
    c. Sodium chloride
    d. Methylparaben

13. Which of the following statements is correct relevant to ester-type local anesthetic agents?
    a. They are manufactured in only one preparation, which is a combination of procaine and benzocaine
    b. They should be administered to patients who have atypical plasma cholinesterase
    c. They have been withdrawn from the US market since January 1996
    d. Their preparation includes methylparaben as a preservative to prolong their shelf life

14. Besides the health status of the patient, what is the most important consideration in choosing an anesthetic?
    a. The duration of time that the patient needs anesthesia
    b. Potential post-treatment discomfort
    c. The patient's preference
    d. The patient's pain threshold

15. What is a safe limit to the number of cartridges of mepivacaine 2% administered to a child of approximately 50 lb?
    a. 2
    b. 4
    c. 5
    d. 7

16. Which type of injection is preferred if hemostasis is a primary consideration for the use of anesthesia?
    a. Field block
    b. Extraoral nerve block
    c. Nerve block
    d. Local infiltration

17. Which anesthetic solution is the **most** appropriate for a 1-hour root planing appointment on a patient with a confirmed hyperthyroid condition?
    a. Lidocaine 2% with 1:50,000 epinephrine
    b. Prilocaine 4%, with 1:200,000 epinephrine
    c. Bupivacaine 0.5% with 1:200,000 epinephrine
    d. Lidocaine 2% without epinephrine

18. Which anesthetic is *most* appropriate to administer to a patient requiring periodontal surgery on teeth 17 to 21?
    a. Citanest plain
    b. 3% Carbocaine
    c. 2% Xylocaine
    d. Marcaine

19. Your patient has chronic adult periodontitis with moderate bone loss. He has extremely sensitive root surfaces and spontaneous hemorrhaging around teeth 12, 13, and 4 with very little detectable calculus deposit. Debridement in that area will take you approximately 15 minutes to perform. He has no medical history complications. What is the most appropriate anesthetic agent to administer?
    a. Carbocaine 2%, 1:20,000
    b. Carbocaine 3%
    c. Xylocaine 2%, 1:100,000
    d. Xylocaine 2%, plain
    e. Marcaine 0.5%

20. How many cartridges of Carbocaine 2% may be administered to a 100-lb healthy woman before reaching her MRD?
    a. 8.3 cartridges
    b. 5.5 cartridges
    c. 11.1 cartridges
    d. 5.0 cartridges
    e. 2.2 cartridges

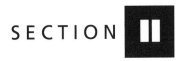

Injections

Information from the Nerve and Technique Summary Charts is compiled from assorted references including these key sources: Auger (2005), Jastek, Yageila, and Donaldson (1995), Evers and Haegerstam (1990), Hiatt and Gartener (2002), Malamed (2004), Lipp (1993)

Nerve Summary Chart

The following summarizes the branches of the trigeminal nerve that are particularly significant in dental pain control:

NERVE	MUCOSA	TEETH
V_2: Maxillary Division		
1. *Pterygopalatine branch*		
a. Nasopalatine	Lingual gingiva of maxillary incisors	
b. Anterior (greater) palatine	All hard palate except lingual gingiva of maxillary incisors	
2. *Infraorbital branch*		
a. Posterior superior alveolar (PSA)	Buccal: maxillary gingiva in molar region	Maxillary molars (except mesiobuccal, root of first molar)
b. Middle superior alveolar (MSA)	Buccal: maxillary gingiva in premolar region	Maxillary premolars and mesiobuccal root of first molar
c. Anterior superior alveolar (ASA)	Facial gingiva of maxillary anteriors	Maxillary anteriors
V_3: Mandibular Division		
1. Long buccal	Cheek and buccal gingiva in molar region	
2. Inferior alveolar, including two terminal branches:	Buccal gingiva from premolars to midline, mucosa, and skin of lower lip	All mandibular teeth in quadrant
a. Mental (terminal branch)	(Buccal gingiva from premolars to midline, mucosa, and skin of lower lip)	
b. Incisive (terminal branch)		(Teeth from premolars through central)
3. Lingual	All mandibular lingual gingiva in quadrant, floor of mouth, and anterior two thirds of tongue	

Innervation Diagram

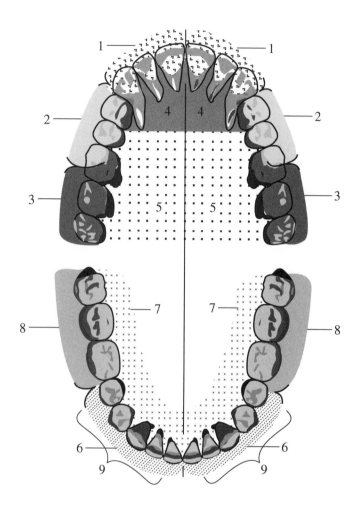

KEY TO INNERVATION DIAGRAM:

1. Anterior Superior Alveolar Nerve $\Big\}$ infraorbital
2. Middle Superior Alveolar Nerve
3. Posterior Superior Alveolar Nerve
4. Nasopalatine Nerve
5. Anterior (greater) Palatine Nerve
6. Inferior Alveolar Nerve: soft tissues of #9 in one quadrant and all of the teeth in that quadrant
7. Lingual Nerve
8. Buccal Nerve
9. Mental: Buccal/Facial Tissues Only
   Incisive: Teeth Only

NOTE: this diagram is also available for downloading/printing in color on the CD ROM.

Technique Summary Chart: Maxillary Injections

	INFILTRATION	ASA	MSA	INFRAORBITAL	PSA	GREATER PALATINE	NASO-PALATINE
Branch of trigeminal nerve	Large terminal nerve endings	Anterior superior alveolar (ASA) branch of infraorbital nerve (V$_2$)	Middle superior alveolar (MSA) branch of infraorbital nerve (V$_2$)	ASA, MSA, inferior palpebral, lateral nasal, and superior labial (branches of infraorbital nerve)	Posterior superior alveolar (PSA) maxillary division (V$_2$)	Greater (or anterior) palatine, branch of pterygopalatine nerve (V$_2$)	Naso-palatine nerve, branch of ptery-gopalatine nerve (V$_2$)
Area anes-thetized (teeth and soft tissue)	Tooth, periosteum and buccal soft tissue in entire area innervated by that nerve branch	Field block that includes maxillary central, lat-eral, cuspid, periosteum, and facial soft tissue of same area (to midline)	Field block that includes maxillary premolars and MB root of max. first molar, periosteum and buccal soft tissue of same area; absent in a large percentage of the population	Max. central to MB root of first molar, periosteum, buccal soft tissue of same area, lower eyelid, lateral aspect of nose, upper lip	Third, second, first maxillary molars (except MB root of first permanent molar if MSA is present); periosteum and buccal soft tissue of same area	No teeth; hard palate and lingual tissue distal to canine and medial to midline	No teeth; anterior third of hard palate; lingual tissues from canine to canine
Needle	25, 27, or 30 short	25, 27, or 30 short	25, 27 or 30 short	25 or 27 long; 27 short for small patient	25 or 27 short	25, 27, or 30 short	25, 27, or 30 short
Landmarks	Mucobuccal fold above tooth being anes-thetized	Canine fossae, located between lateral and canine	Malar process (zygomatic strut); max. premolars	Infraorbital notch; infraorbital foramen	Zygomatic buttress/malar strut, maxillary tuberosity, ala of nose, corner of mouth	Vertical and horizontal processes of maxillae and pala-tine bones	Max. centrals, incisive papilla

(continued)

	INFILTRATION	ASA	MSA	INFRAORBITAL	PSA	GREATER PALATINE	NASO-PALATINE
Insertion/penetration site	Height of mucobuccal fold apical to tooth being anesthetized	Height of mucobuccal fold mesial to root of canine at canine fossa	Height of mucobuccal fold over max. second premolar	Height of mucobuccal fold over max. first premolar	Height of mucobuccal fold in concavity distal to zygomatic buttress, distal of second molar, 45-degree angle from occlusal plane	Greater palatine foramen and junction of max. alveolar process and palatine bone; to either side of incisive papilla	next to base of incisive papilla
Approximate depth of penetration[a]	4–6 mm, $1/4$ in.	4–6 mm, $1/4$ in.	4–10 mm, $1/4$–$1/2$ in.	$1/2$ length of long needle ($3/4$ in., 16 mm)	$3/4$ in., 16 mm (3–4 mm from hub of short needle)	$1/8$–$1/4$ in. (usually 3–6 mm)	$1/8$–$1/4$ in. (usually 3–6 mm)
Deposition/target site	Apex of tooth to be anesthetized	mesial to the apex of maxillary canine	over apex of second premolar	Directly over infraorbital foramen	Posterior, superior, and medial to maxillary tuberosity; 45-degree angle to occlusal plane; 45-degree angle to mid-saggital plane	Slightly anterior to greater (anterior) palatine foramen	Over the incisive foramen; one injection will anesthetize both right and left nasopalatine nerves.
Volume of anesthetic[a]	1.0–1.8 mL ($1/2$–1 cartridge)	1.0–1.2 mL ($1/2$–$2/3$ cartridge)	1.0–1.2 mL ($1/2$–$2/3$ cartridge)	1.2–1.5 mL ($2/3$–$3/4$ cartridge)	1–1.8 mL ($3/4$–1 cartridge)	0.45 to 0.6 mL ($1/4$–$1/3$ cartridge)	0.2–0.45 mL ($1/8$–$1/4$ cartridge)
Potential complications/additional considerations	Not effective on mandible due to dense cortical bone; Not suitable for large areas because of multiple needle insertions and increase in total volume of local anesthetic	Pain if periosteum is scraped Ballooning of tissue possible; Often central innervation overlap; may require additional infiltration over central	Pain if periosteum is scraped; Ballooning of tissue possible; Large percentage of population does not have MSA	Psychological fear of eye injury, palpation may be uncomfortable, or difficulty defining landmarks	Mandibular anesthesia if anesthetic is deposited too far laterally; No bony landmark, risk of hematoma; hemorrhage, may be problem for some patients; May require second injection for MB root of first molar	No hemostasis except in injection area	Necrosis of soft tissue from vasoconstrictor is possible; No hemostasis except in injection area; Potentially most traumatic injection

[a]The depth of penetration and the volume of anesthetic will ultimately depend on the procedure being performed and individual anatomy.

Note: This chart is also available in downloadable format on the CD.

Technique Summary Chart: Mandibular Injections

	INFERIOR ALVEOLAR AND LINGUAL	BUCCAL	MENTAL	INCISIVE	GOW GATES
Branch of trigeminal nerve	Inferior alveolar nerve: branch of posterior root of mandibular (V_3) Lingual nerve: branch of posterior root of mandibular (V_3)	Long buccal nerve, branch of anterior root of mandibular (V_3)	Terminal branch of the inferior alveolar nerve	Terminal branch of the inferior alveolar nerve	Entire V_3 mandibular division (inferior alveolar, mental, incisive, lingual, buccal, mylohyoid, auriculotemporal)
Area Anesthetized (teeth and/or soft tissue)	Inferior alveolar nerve: mandibular teeth to midline (molars, premolars, cuspid, central, lateral); body of mandible, all buccal soft tissue except buccal area of molars, Lingual nerve: no teeth; lingual gingiva of mandibular quadrant (central to third molar), anterior two thirds of tongue, floor of mouth. The lingual nerve is commonly anesthetized during the inferior alveolar injection but can be done separately	No teeth; Soft tissues and periosteum buccal to mandibular molars	No teeth; Buccal soft tissues from mental foramen to midline and the soft tissues of the lower lip and chin	Teeth anterior to the mental foramen (premolars, cuspid, lateral, central)	Entire quadrant on mandible: all teeth, facial and lingual gingiva, soft tissues of lower lip and chin, anterior two thirds of tongue, floor of mouth, auriculotemporal area
Needle	25 or 27 long	25 or 27 long because it follows inferior alveolar	25 or 27 short	25 or 27 short	25 or 27 long
Landmarks	Coronoid notch, pterygomandibular raphe, occlusal plane of mandibular premolar teeth, and commissure on contralateral side	External oblique ridge and second molar; retromolar fossa	Mental foramen-usually located between the two premolars; however, may be either anterior or posterior to this site	Same as mental; palpate foramen by placing finger in mucobuccal fold in first molar area; move it anteriorly until you feel the bone become irregular; radiographs are helpful	Extraoral: intertragic notch, corner of mouth Intraoral: mesiolingual cusp of maxillary second molar

(continued)

	INFERIOR ALVEOLAR AND LINGUAL	BUCCAL	MENTAL	INCISIVE	GOW GATES
Insertion/ penetration site	Medial to internal and external oblique ridges; height of coronoid notch; lateral to pterygomandibular raphe The lingual nerve will be anesthetized during the same insertion for IA injection	Mucobuccal fold distal and buccal to last molar; parallel with occlusal plane	Mental foramen usually between apices of first and second premolars, mucobuccal fold	Mental foramen usually between apices of first and second premolars, mucobuccal fold	Intertragic notch, corner of mouth Height: mesiolingual cusp of maxillary second molar Penetration: distal to maxillary second molar
Approximate depth of penetration[a]	Inferior alveolar: 20–25 mm, $2/3$–$3/4$ length of long needle Lingual: $1/2$ distance of inferior alveolar	3–6 mm ($1/8$–$1/4$ in.)	4–6 mm ($1/8$–$1/4$ in.)	4–6 mm ($1/8$–$1/4$ in.)	Average 25 mm to $3/4$ length of long needle
Deposition/ target site	Inferior alveolar: directly above mandibular foramen Lingual: Half the distance to mandibular foramen at lingual nerve	Medial to external oblique ridge; distal and buccal to last molar	Directly over the mental foramen	Directly over mental foramen; use finger pressure to direct solution into the foramen	Neck of condyle
Volume of anesthetic[a]	Inferior alveolar: 1.5–1.8 mL ($3/4$–1 cartridge) Lingual: 0.25–0.5 mL ($1/8$ cartridge)	0.25–0.5 mL ($1/8$ cartridge)	0.5–1.0 mL ($1/3$–$1/2$ cartridge)	0.5–1.0 mL ($1/3$–$1/2$ cartridge)	1.8 mL (1 cartridge)
Potential complications/additional considerations	Too far medially: medial pterygoid muscle; trismus Too deep: facial nerve paralysis if anesthetic is deposited in parotid gland Wide area anesthesia; lower lip anesthesia; Warn patients not to bite lip or tongue; Shocking pain if lingual nerve touched	Uncomfortable if needle contacts periosteum	Possibility of hematoma	Possibility of hematoma; Incisive nerve blocks teeth only; however, mental nerve will be anesthetized incidentally when this injection is administered	Warn patient not to bite lip or tongue Longer onset time, wide area of anesthesia, learning curve for operator

[a]The depth of penetration and the volume of anesthetic will ultimately depend on the procedure being performed and individual anatomy.

Note: This chart is also available in downloadable format on the CD

Alternative Materials, Devices, and Techniques Available in the United States

PRODUCT	BRAND NAMES	MANUFACTURER
Eutectic mixture of local anesthetics	EMLA Oraquix	Dentsply Dentsply
Topical anesthetic patches	Dentipatch Benzocaine Patches	Noven Premier
Electronic dental anesthesia	Cedeta Mk3	Cedeta Dental International, Inc.
Computer-controlled systems	CompuDent Comfort Control Syringe	Milestone Scientific Dentsply
Periodontal ligament anesthesia (PDL) syringes	Pen Type Gun Type SoftJect	Septodont and others Miltex Henke (Germany)
Intraosseous anesthesia systems	Stabident X-tip IntraFlow	Fairfax Dental Dentsply International Intravantage, Inc.
Carbonated local anesthetic	None	Must mix with individual cartridges
Safety syringes/needles	Safemate Simple Safety Plus System Scoop Cap Ultrasafe Syringes 1 Shot Safety Syringes	Septodont Septodont Benco Dental Safety Syringes, Inc. Sultan Chemicals

These are some brands available from US manufacturers in 2006; others also may be available at this time. Review literature and catalogs for updated products.

SECTION II LEARNING ACTIVITIES

1. Review the following diagrams. Identify each structure by writing in the appropriate name on the corresponding blank line. After indicating your answers, refer to the answer key to check your responses.

Nerves

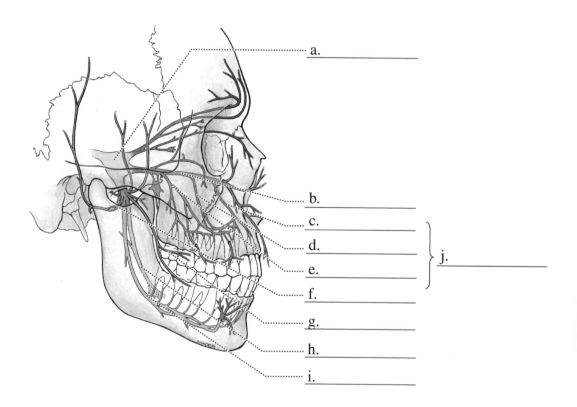

a. _____

b. _____

c. _____

d. _____ ⎫

e. _____ ⎬ j. _____

f. _____ ⎭

g. _____

h. _____

i. _____

Mandibular Anatomy

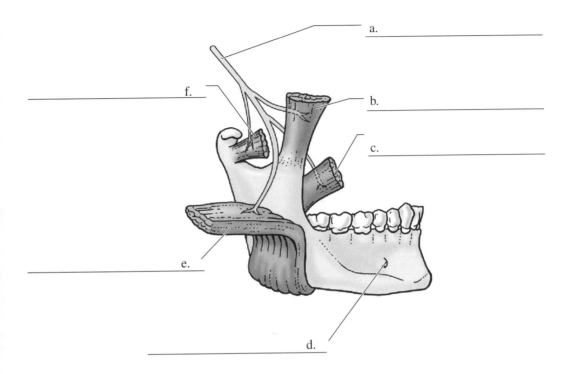

a. _____

b. _____

c. _____

d. _____

e. _____

f. _____

Blood supply

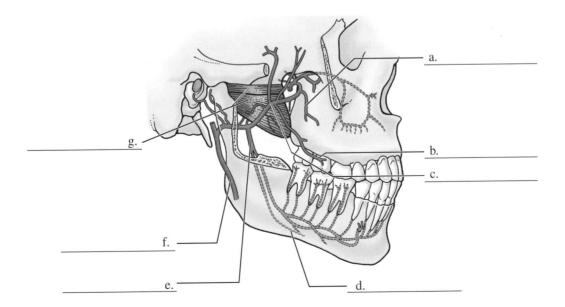

a. _____

b. _____

c. _____

d. _____

e. _____

f. _____

g. _____

2. Identify the following structures on a skull, noting the relevance of each structure to the corresponding injection(s) in that area:

STRUCTURE	NOTES
Superior orbital fissure	
Foramen rotundum	
Foramen ovale	
Pterygopalatine fossa	
Posterior superior foramina	
Infraorbital notch	
Intraorbital foramen	
Floor of orbit	
Zygomatic bone/strut/buttress and arch	
Maxillary tuberosity	
Canine eminence	
Greater palatine foramen	
Lesser palatine foramen	
Incisive foramen	
Mandibular foramen	
Condyle	
Coronoid process	
Coronoid notch	
Ramus	
Alveolar process	
Palatine process of palatal bones	
Palatine process of maxilla	

3. Look at the document on the CD entitled *Technique Errors*. The presentation demonstrates common technique errors that frequently occur during the administration of local anesthesia. View each image, determine the injection being given, and establish ways to correct the errors. After identifying the problem(s) on the first slide, click to view the subsequent slide, which will confirm the errors and demonstrate a more appropriate technique.

4. Review the current literature and identify advantages and disadvantages of the following alternate techniques and/or devices:

Intraosseous anesthesia (e.g., IntraFlow®, Stabident®)

Computer-controlled local anesthesia systems (e.g., CompuDent®, ComfortControl®)

Electronic dental anesthesia (e.g., Cedeta®)

Alternative topical anesthetic products (e.g., Oraqix®, DentiPatch®)

PDL syringes (SoftJect® Citoject)

5. In preparation for clinical experience, or to review details for each injection, complete the Local Anesthesia Study Guide Guides by filling in the relevant information for each of the injections listed. Use the information presented in Section II.3 on the CD-ROM to assist you if needed.

LOCAL ANESTHESIA STUDY GUIDE: MANDIBULAR INJECTIONS

	INFERIOR ALVEOLAR	BUCCAL	MENTAL	INCISIVE	GOW GATES
Nerve anesthetized:					
Teeth/hard tissue anesthetized:					
Soft tissue anesthetized:					
Recommended needle:					
Landmarks:					
Site of needle penetration:					
Deposition area (target area):					
Depth of needle penetration:					
Amount of recommended anesthetic solution:					
Potential complications:					

LOCAL ANESTHESIA STUDY GUIDE: MAXILLARY INJECTIONS

	INFILTRATION	INFRAORBITAL	PSA	GREATER PALATINE	NASOPALATINE
Nerve anesthetized:					
Teeth/hard tissue anesthetized:					
Soft tissue anesthetized:					
Recommended needle:					
Landmarks:					
Site of needle penetration:					
Deposition area (target area):					
Depth of needle penetration:					
Amount of recommended anesthetic solution:					
Potential complications:					

6. Use the sample Local Anesthesia Evaluation Form to self-assess your injection technique. Choose your two most challenging injections (or use the inferior alveolar and PSA) to assess.

LOCAL ANESTHESIA COMPETENCY EVALUATION

Evaluation Rating Scale

N = Not applicable

0 = Unsatisfactory   Any **0** should be repeated

1 = Needs improvement

2 = Satisfactory   INJECTION_____

PERFORMANCE CRITERIA	RATING			
1. Places needle in cartridge properly, engages harpoon	N	0	1	2
2. Tests set-up prior to use	N	0	1	2
3. Aligns bevel of needle appropriately	N	0	1	2
4. Aligns large window toward operator	N	0	1	2
5. Positions patient properly	N	0	1	2
6. Arranges adequate lighting and visibility	N	0	1	2
7. Visually and by palpation, locates and identifies the landmarks	N	0	1	2
8. Wipes area with gauze; applies topical anesthetic for minimum of 1–2 min	N	0	1	2
9. Grasps movable soft tissues securely to achieve sufficient stability and visibility	N	0	1	2
*10. Establishes a fulcrum	N	0	1	2
*11. Penetrates tissue at desired insertion site	N	0	1	2
*12. Follows correct pathway of insertion	N	0	1	2
*13. Proceeds to proper depth for injection and indicates site of deposition	N	0	1	2
*14. Aspirates prior to depositing solution	N	0	1	2
*15. Injects slowly and with control using proper dose	N	0	1	2
16. Maintains safe and aseptic technique	N	0	1	2
17. Manages patient in a manner that minimizes anxiety and discomfort and promotes safety (i.e., prepares patient, keeps needle out of patient's sight, reassures patient throughout procedure, avoids unnecessary relocation of needle, etc.)	N	0	1	2
18. Achieves anesthesia appropriate for given clinical situation	N	0	1	2
19. Recaps and discards needle according to OSHA standards	N	0	1	2
20. Accurately records procedures on patient treatment record	N	0	1	2

*Critical Error: Must receive a **2** before passing competency.

ANSWER KEY TO DIAGRAMS IN QUESTION 1.

NERVES	MANDIBULAR ANATOMY	ARTERIAL BLOOD SUPPLY
a. Trigeminal ganglion	a. Mandibular nerve	a. PSA
b. Infraorbital	b. Temporalis muscle	b. Buccal
c. Anterior	c. Medial pterygoid muscle	c. Maxillary
d. Middle	d. Mental foramen	d. Branch to mylohyoid
e. Posterior	e. Masseter muscle	e. Inferior alveolar
f. Auriculotemporal	f. Lateral pterygoid muscle	f. External carotid
g. Buccal		g. Lateral pterygoid muscle
h. Lingual		
i. Inferior alveolar		
j. Superior alveolar nerves		

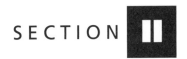

Injections/Quizzes

Trigeminal Nerve

SECTION **2-1**

1. View the diagram of the cranium below.
   a–c. Label the fissure and foramina identified.
   d–f. Name the branch/division of the trigeminal nerve that goes through each of the above.

   Fissure/foramen *corresponds* with   Branch of trigeminal

   a._____   d._____

   b._____   e._____

   c._____   f._____

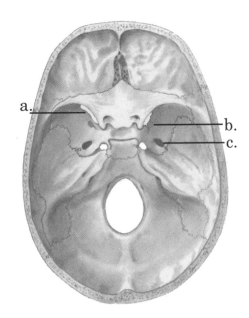

2. The cell bodies of origin of the afferent fibers of the fifth cranial nerve are located:
   a. Within the cerebral cortex
   b. Within the pons
   c. Within the trigeminal ganglion
   d. None of the above

3. The teeth and/or tissues innervated by the middle superior alveolar nerve are:
   a. Maxillary third molar; second molar; and distobuccal and lingual roots of first molar, as well as the buccal gingiva in that region
   b. Maxillary third molar; second molar; and distobuccal and lingual roots of first molar, as well as the lingual gingiva in that region
   c. Maxillary third, second, first molars with associated buccal and lingual tissue
   d. Maxillary first premolar; second premolar; and mesiobuccal root of first molar, as well as the buccal gingiva in that region
   e. Maxillary first premolar; second premolar; and mesiobuccal root of first molar, as well as the lingual gingiva in that region
   f. Maxillary first premolar, second premolar, and mesiobuccal root of first molar with associated buccal and lingual gingiva

4. The incisive nerve is a terminal branch of the:
   a. Mental nerve
   b. Inferior alveolar nerve
   c. Nasopalatine nerve
   d. Greater palatine nerve
   e. Infraorbital nerve

5. What is the position of the lingual nerve in relation to the inferior alveolar nerve?
   a. Anterior and lateral
   b. Anterior and medial
   c. Posterior and lateral
   d. Posterior and medial

6–9. View the diagram of the mandible below. Label the three nerves, as well as the other structure that is identified.

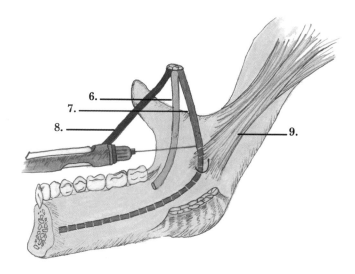

6. _____

7. _____

8. _____

9. _____

10. **Matching:** Match the area with the nerve innervating that area, assuming normal nerve placement. There may be more than one answer. Answers may be used more than once.

_____dental pulp, #2   a. Nasopalatine (NP)

_____dental pulp, #12   b. MSA (middle superior alveolar)

_____dental pulp, #7   c. Incisive

_____lingual gingiva, #7   d. Mental

_____lingual gingiva, #14   e. Anterior (greater) palatine

_____buccal gingiva, #22   f. PSA (posterior superior alveolar)

_____dental pulp, #24   g. ASA (anterior superior alveolar)

11. The incisive nerve is a branch of the infraorbital nerve, exiting onto the hard palate through the incisive foramen.
    a. True
    b. False

12. What teeth and tissues are innervated by the inferior alveolar nerve?
    a. All mandibular molars and premolars as well as the buccal tissue in that region.
    b. All mandibular teeth from the premolars to the midline as well as the buccal tissue from the premolars to the midline.
    c. All mandibular teeth from the third molar to the midline as well as the buccal tissue in the molar region.
    d. All mandibular teeth from the premolars to the midline as well as the buccal tissue from the third molar to the midline.
    e. All mandibular teeth from the third molar to the midline as well as the buccal tissue from the premolars to the midline.

13. The teeth and/or tissues innervated by the PSA nerve are maxillary third molar; second molar; and distobuccal and lingual roots of first molar, as well as the buccal gingiva in that region.
    a. True
    b. False

14. The buccinator nerve originates on the lateral surface of the skull in a fan shape.
    a. True
    b. False

15. The medial pterygoid muscle inserts at the angle of the mandible—the lateral surface.
    a. True
    b. False

16. The inferior alveolar nerve passes through the mandibular foramen.
    a. True
    b. False

17. The facial gingiva of tooth #22 is innervated by a terminal branch of the inferior alveolar nerve.
    a. True
    b. False

18. The nerve(s) whose main trunk exits the cranium through the foramen rotundum is:
    a. PSA
    b. MSA
    c. ASA
    d. Greater (anterior) palatine
    e. All of the above

19. Branches of the mandibular artery supply the mandibular teeth.
    a. True
    b. False

20. The facial gingiva of tooth 30 is innervated by the inferior alveolar nerve.
    a. True
    b. False

21. To completely anesthetize tooth #15 and all tissues, you will need to block the PSA, MSA, and AP (anterior palatine).
    a. True
    b. False

Armamentarium Self-Test

SECTION **2-2**

1. Which of the following gauge numbers indicates the needle with the largest lumen?
   a. 23
   b. 25
   c. 27
   d. 30

2. How much solution is contained in dental anesthetic cartridges manufactured in the US?
   a. 0.18 cc
   b. 0.018 mL
   c. 1.8 mL
   d. 18.0 cc
   e. 1.8 cc
   f. c and e

3. The hemostat should always be included on the local anesthetic tray setup in the event that a needle should break. Needle breakage is a fairly common occurrence, particularly at the hub of the needle.
   a. Both sentences are true
   b. Both sentences are false
   c. The first sentence is true; the second sentence is false
   d. The first sentence is false; the second sentence is true

4. Anesthetic cartridges should be autoclaved after opening a canister or blister package to ensure sterility.
   a. True
   b. False

5. What is an advantage of using a 25-gauge rather than a 30-gauge needle?
   a. Ease of penetration
   b. Ease of aspiration
   c. Decreased deflection
   d. Increased patient comfort
   e. b and c

6. What is the approximate length of a long needle?
   a. 20–21 mm
   b. 22–24 mm
   c. 25–27 mm
   d. 28–30 mm
   e. >30 mm

7–11. Label the parts of this syringe by matching the letter from the list of parts with the number by each arrow.

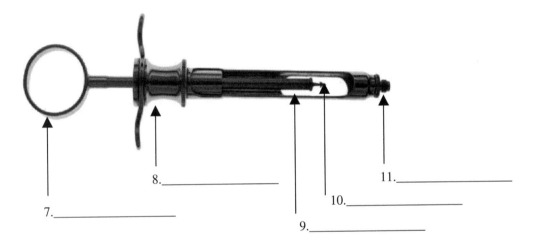

8._____   11._____

                                  10._____

7._____

                        9._____

   a. Spring lock
   b. Finger grip (or spool finger grip)
   c. Large window
   d. Adapter
   e. Harpoon
   f. Bevel
   g. Small window
   h. Thumb ring

12. Is the syringe pictured above an aspirating or a non-aspirating syringe?

_____

13–15. Label the parts of this cartridge by matching the letter from the list of parts with the number by each arrow.

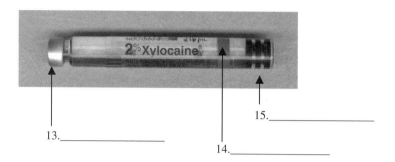

15._____

13._____

14._____

    a. Rubber stopper
    b. Glass cylinder
    c. Aluminum cap
    d. Adapter
    e. Rubber diaphragm
    f. Bevel
    g. Color-coded band indicating expiration date

16–18. Needles:

Needles:

A

B

16. What gauge needle is shown in A (blue cap)? _____

17. What gauge needle is shown in B (yellow cap)? _____

18. Is B a long or short needle? _____

19. What color cap does a 25-gauge needle have?

20. How often should disposable needles be changed? _____

Technique

1. Which of the following types of injections anesthetizes the smallest area:
   a. Field block
   b. Nerve block
   c. Infiltration

2. An inferior alveolar injection is considered a:
   a. Nerve block
   b. Field block
   c. Local infiltration
   d. None of the above

3. It is more important for the patient to be more comfortable than the operator during an injection since anesthesia can be so stress inducing.
   a. True
   b. False

4. A positive aspiration indicates:
   a. You have inserted into an area of infection
   b. You put positive pressure on the thumb ring
   c. The tip of the needle may be within a blood vessel
   d. Reappointing the patient for another time
   e. c and d

5. The target area (deposition site) of the posterior superior alveolar nerve block is:
   a. The foramen posterior and superior to the maxillary second (and/or third) molar
   b. The maxillary bone superior to the apex of the maxillary second premolar
   c. The infraorbital foramen
   d. The height of the mucobuccal fold of the second molar
   e. None of the above

6. While providing pressure anesthesia during an anterior palatine injection:
   a. The needle is slipped through the cotton applicator stick and into the tissue
   b. An applicator stick should be positioned just posterior to the foramen
   c. Steady, firm pressure causes the incisive papilla to blanch
   d. An applicator stick placed directly over the foramen may be used to anesthetize the area prior to needle insertion

7. During the insertion phase of an injection, the patient complains of a momentary sensation of an electric shock. You have most likely:
   a. Contacted the nerve sheath with the needle
   b. Severed a small nerve fiber with the needle
   c. Injected too rapidly
   d. Injected before the topical anesthetic has taken effect

8. Which of the following is *not* a possible use of a 2 × 2 gauze sponge while administering a local anesthetic?
   a. To dry the injection site prior to applying the topical anesthetic
   b. To wipe the needle prior to the injection
   c. To remove the topical anesthetic from the injection site prior to insertion
   d. To absorb any hemorrhage from the injection site until hemostasis is achieved

9. Which injection technique decreases systemic absorption of local anesthetic?
   a. Injecting rapidly
   b. Injecting slowly
   c. Selecting a local anesthetic without epinephrine
   d. Depositing the solution intramuscularly
   e. Aspirating prior to reaching the target area of the injection

10. What condition is avoided by aspiration prior to deposition of a local anesthetic?
    a. Intravascular injection
    b. Vascular injury
    c. Permanent anesthesia of the area
    d. Damage to the periosteum of the bone

11. Where is the insertion site for the inferior alveolar nerve block?
    a. Medial to the pterygoid fossa, lateral to the pterygomandibular raphe, at the height of the occlusal plane
    b. Medial to the internal oblique ridge, lateral to the pterygomandibular raphe, the height of the occlusal plane
    c. Medial to the pterygoid fossa, lateral to the pterygomandibular raphe, at the height of the coronoid notch
    d. Medial to the internal oblique ridge, lateral to the pterygomandibular raphe, at the height of the coronoid notch

12. Where should the needle tip be located when depositing anesthetic for the inferior alveolar nerve block?
    a. Slightly anterior to the mandibular foramen
    b. Slightly posterior to the mandibular foramen
    c. Slightly superior to the mandibular foramen
    d. Slightly inferior to the mandibular foramen

13. Upon administration of a right inferior alveolar injection with 1 carpule of anesthetic, the dental hygienist discovers that the patient does not have profound anesthesia. Prior to reinjecting, she evaluates the patient's occlusion and notes that the patient has class III occlusion. Which of the following changes in technique is most appropriate to achieve profound anesthesia for this patient?
    a. No changes in technique are necessary; readminister injection in same location
    b. Select a penetration site 1 cm lateral to the original injection site
    c. Select a penetration site 1 cm lower than the original injection site
    d. Select a penetration site 1 cm higher than the original injection site

14. Deposition of anesthetic solution should never exceed:
    a. $^1/_2$ cartridge per minute
    b. 1 cartridge per minute
    c. 1.8 mL per 30 seconds
    d. $^1/_4$ cartridge per minute

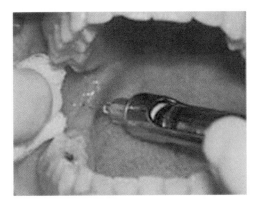

15. Look at the photo. Assuming normal nerve placement and a successful injection, what teeth and tissue are being anesthetized with this injection?
    1. All mandibular teeth from the third molar to the midline
    2. Mandibular molars and premolars only
    3. All mandibular lingual gingiva from the second premolar to the midline
    4. All facial tissue from mandibular third molar to the midline
    5. Buccal tissue in mandibular molar region
    6. Buccal tissue from mandibular second premolar to midline

    Answer:
    a. 1, 3, 4, and 5
    b. 2, 3, and 5
    c. 1, 3, and 5
    d. 1, 4, and 5
    e. 1, 3, and 6
    f. 2 and 4 only
    g. 1 and 5 only
    h. 1 and 3 only
    i. 1 and 6 only

16. One landmark essential to the anesthetize of the lingual gingiva of the maxillary anterior teeth is:
    a. Nasopalatine foramen
    b. Greater palatine foramen
    c. Premolar teeth
    d. Incisive foramen

17. Facial nerve paralysis is most commonly caused by introduction of local anesthetic into the parotid gland during which injection?
    a. Posterior superior alveolar
    b. Infraorbital
    c. Inferior alveolar
    d. Nasopalatine
    e. Anterior palatine

18. With which injection does a hematoma most commonly occur?
    a. Posterior superior alveolar
    b. Inferior alveolar
    c. Middle superior alveolar
    d. Anterior palatine
    e. Anterior superior alveolar

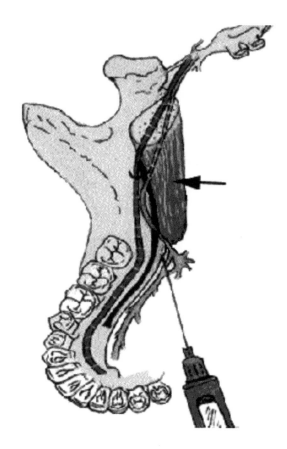

19. View the photo. To what structure is the arrow pointing?

    _____

20. What is the name of the depression along the anterior border of the ramus that is an anatomical landmark for an inferior alveolar nerve block injection?
    a. Mandibular sulcus
    b. Pterygoid fossa
    c. Condylar notch
    d. Coronoid notch

21. Which of the following anatomical structures would most commonly pose a potential hazard during the posterior superior alveolar nerve block injection?
    a. Masseter muscle
    b. Pterygoid venous plexus
    c. Parotid gland
    d. Buccal branch of the facial nerve

22. In what instance should a clinician respond to a positive aspiration by removing the syringe, changing the cartridge, and redoing the procedure?
   a. The patient is moving too much
   b. The dental hygienist cannot clearly see that the aspiration is negative
   c. The patient has hemophilia
   d. The needle hits bone

23. What is the correct procedure to anesthetize the long buccal nerve?
   a. Withdraw the needle halfway from the mandibular foramen, aspirate, and deposit
   b. Insert in the buccal mucosa at the apex of the premolars to cover the bevel, aspirate, and deposit
   c. Palpate the external oblique, insert medially to it, at the height of the distobuccal cusp of the last molar, aspirate, and deposit
   d. Palpate the external oblique, insert laterally to it, aspirate, and deposit

24. Where is the insertion site for a posterior superior alveolar nerve block?
   a. Anterior to the zygomatic process
   b. Posterior to the zygomatic process
   c. Distal to the maxillary tuberosity
   d. Medial to the maxillary tuberosity

25. Where is the correct injection site for the MSA (middle superior alveolar) field block?
   a. Above the apex of the first premolar
   b. Above the apex of the second premolar
   c. Between the first and second premolars and above the apex of both teeth
   d. Between the lateral and cuspid and above the apex of both teeth

Selection of Injections

S E C T I O N **2-4**

1. Which statement is *false* concerning anesthetizing a patient with an abscess of #20.
   a. Tooth #20 may be difficult to anesthetize with an incisive nerve block because the acidic environment around the apex of the tooth reduces the availability of local anesthetic free base.
   b. Tooth #20 may be difficult to anesthetize with an incisive nerve block because the acidic environment around the apex of the tooth increases the availability of local anesthetic free base.
   c. The tissue around #20 may have increased vascularity and edema, which may dilute the concentration of local anesthetic and prevent impulse blockade if an incisive nerve block is administered.
   d. Tooth #20 may be effectively anesthetized by using the inferior alveolar nerve block because the site of infection is located away from the local anesthetic deposition site.

2. In what instance(s) should a clinician give the long buccal nerve block?
   a. Routinely after an inferior alveolar nerve block
   b. Only when the buccal tissues of the mandibular molars need anesthesia
   c. For greater patient comfort while scaling facial aspect throughout the mandibular quadrant
   d. Instead of the inferior alveolar nerve block when curettage of the mandibular premolars is planned

3. A clinician determines that a patient has a periodontal-endodontic abscess on the lingual aspect of tooth #13. A dental hygienist is to curet the abscess. Which nerves require anesthesia for this procedure?
   a. Anterior superior alveolar, nasopalatine
   b. Middle superior alveolar, nasopalatine
   c. Anterior superior, greater palatine
   d. Middle superior alveolar, greater palatine

4. What nerve block should a clinician give to obtain anesthesia of the labial soft tissue associated with teeth #26 and #27?
   a. Lingual
   b. Incisive
   c. Mental
   d. Long buccal

5. For most mandibular teeth, infiltration anesthesia is:
   a. Impractical because of the density of the bone of the mandible
   b. Not practical because of the distance and location of the nerves from the cortical plate
   c. Impractical because of the porosity of the bone of the mandible
   d. Used most commonly

6. A patient complains of sensitivity to heat, cold, and pressure. Examination of the radiograph reveals a radiolucency around the apex of tooth #15. Which of the following is the best injection(s) to complete anesthesia of that tooth?
   a. PSA
   b. MSA
   c. Infraorbital block
   d. Local infiltration above 15
   e. a and b above

7. You have given the injection selected in question 6 above, plus some additional anesthesia above the root in that area. The patient continues to have discomfort. The *most* likely reason for inadequate anesthesia is:
   a. The capillaries are in a hypotonic state because of the abscess
   b. There is increased pressure on the nerves due to the swelling
   c. The acidity produced by inflammation inhibits the action of the anesthetic
   d. The anesthetic has been diluted by increased fluids in the area

8. Indications for administration of the long buccal nerve block include:
   1. Placement of rubber dam clamp on tooth #18
   2. Removal of Class V caries on the buccal of tooth #19
   3. Placement of a stainless steel matrix band on tooth #20
   4. Soft tissue curettage of buccal gingiva of teeth #19 and #20
   5. Class III restoration of tooth #24 without the use of a clamp

   Answer:
   a. 1, 2, 3
   b. 1, 2, 4
   c. 1 only
   d. 3 only
   e. All of the above

9. If hemostasis is one of the primary considerations for the use of anesthetic, which type of injection is preferred?
   a. Field block
   b. Extraoral nerve block
   c. Nerve block
   d. Local infiltration

10. To extract tooth #17, which injections must be given to anesthetize all pulpal and soft tissue?
    1. PSA
    2. Lingual
    3. Long buccal
    4. Anterior palatine
    5. Inferior alveolar

    Answer
    a. 1, 2
    b. 1, 2, and 3
    c. 1, 4
    d. 2, 5
    e. 2, 3, and 5

Alternative Materials, Devices, and Techniques

S E C T I O N **2-5**

1. Which of the following identifies the TENS techniques of local anesthesia?
   a. Anesthesia is obtained by applying a low-voltage electrical impulse to the target area
   b. The level of anesthesia is controlled by the patient
   c. Not effective for use during an extraction
   d. Placebo effect may play a role in the anesthesia effect
   e. All of the above

2. Which local anesthetic is available in cartridges in the US?
   a. Centrabucridine
   b. Ropivacaine
   c. Articaine
   d. Carbonated local anesthetic
   e. Felypressin

3. Why are carbonated local anesthetics more effective than plain anesthetics?
   a. They reduce inflammation in the area of injection
   b. They increase the number of base molecules available
   c. They increase the number of cation molecules available
   d. They reduce the potential for allergic reactions
   e. a and b

4. Anesthetic patches are effective for approximately how long?
   a. 10 min
   b. 20 min
   c. 30 min
   d. 45 min
   e. 60 min

5. Articaine may be more effective than other anesthetics due to what characteristic?
   a. High protein binding
   b. High pH
   c. Lower concentration of anesthetic agent
   d. a and b
   e. All of the above

6. Which of the following can be used to produce profound topical anesthesia?
   a. EMLA
   b. EDA
   c. Anesthetic patches
   d. TENS
   e. All of the above

7. What is an advantage to using the vasoconstrictor felypressin?
   a. It is better at providing hemorrhage control
   b. It has less effect on the cardiovascular system than other vasoconstrictors
   c. It is produced in concentrations different from those of other vasoconstrictors
   d. a and b
   e. All of the above

8. Which injection technique provides anesthesia to individual teeth?
   a. The Wand®
   b. PDL
   c. Intraosseous (e.g., Stabident)
   d. EMLA
   e. b and c

9. Which needle was specifically manufactured to administer a PDL injection
   a. 25-gauge short
   b. 27-gauge short
   c. 27-gauge ultrashort
   d. 30-gauge short
   e. 30-gauge ultrashort

10. Which injection requires additional equipment (beyond a syringe and needle) to provide anesthesia?
    a. Intraosseous
    b. PDL
    c. The Wand
    d. a and c
    e. All of the above

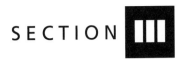

Health History Evaluation and Potential Complications

Sample Health History Form

Medical Alerts:

Answers to the following questions are for our records. This information is confidential and will become part of your permanent dental record.

Please use pen to record information requested within this form.

❏ Mr ❏ Mrs ❏ Ms Name_____

                         (Last)   (First)   (MI)

Social Security Number_____Sex ❏M ❏F

Date of Birth____/____/____   Home Phone Number (_____)_____

Address_____

                      Street   City, State   Zip Code

Employer's Name_____

Employer Phone No_____Ext._____Group No_____

Insurance Name_____ Policy No_____

Name of Person to Notify in Case of an Emergency:

_____

Address_____

Relationship_____Day Phone Number (_____)_____

DENTAL HISTORY   CIRCLE

1. Are you having pain or discomfort at this time?	Yes	No
2. Do you feel nervous about having dental treatment?	Yes	No
3. Have you ever had an upsetting experience in the dental office?	Yes	No
4. Have you noticed any loosening of your teeth?	Yes	No
5. Do you suffer from pain, swelling, or bleeding of your gums?	Yes	No
6. Does food tend to become caught between your teeth?	Yes	No
7. Are you satisfied with the appearance of your teeth?	Yes	No
8. Would it bother you to lose your teeth?	Yes	No

9. Check any of the following that you *have had* or *have* at present.

❑ Teeth extracted

❑ Periodontal (gum) treatment/surgery

❑ Orthodontic treatment

❑ Mouthguard, retainer, partial, or denture

❑ Occlusal equilibration or bite adjustment

❑ Pain/discomfort of the jaw (joint, ear, side of face)

❑ Clicking of the jaw

❑ Difficulty in opening/closing your jaw

❑ Difficulty in chewing

MEDICAL HISTORY   CIRCLE

1. How do you rate your general health?   Good   Fair   Poor

2. Has there been any change in your general health within the past year?	Yes	No
3. Have you been under the care of a medical doctor during the past 2 years? Date of your last physical exam_____	Yes	No
4. Have you ever been hospitalized, or had a serious illness?	Yes	No
5. When you walk up stairs or take a walk, do you ever have to stop because of pain in your chest, shortness of breath, or because you are very tired?	Yes	No
6. Do your ankles swell during the day?	Yes	No
7. Do you require more than two pillows to sleep or do you have an elevated bed?	Yes	No
8. Have you lost or gained more than 10 pounds in the past year? Please record your weight. (Used to determine dosage of local anesthesia if administered.)_____lbs.	Yes	No
9. Are you on a medically recommended diet?	Yes	No
10. Do you have to urinate more than six times a day?	Yes	No
11. Are you frequently thirsty?	Yes	No
12. Does your mouth frequently become dry? If yes, probable cause._____	Yes	No
13. Has your medical doctor ever said you have cancer or a tumor?	Yes	No
14. Are you wearing contact lenses? Soft ___ Hard ___	Yes	No

Women Only:

15. Are you pregnant? Expected delivery date:_____	Yes	No
16. Do you have any problems associated with your menstrual period?	Yes	No
17. Are you nursing?	Yes	No

18. Please check any of the following that you *have had* or *have* at present:

❑ Congestive Heart Failure   ❑ Heart Surgery   ❑ Mitral Valve Prolapse

❑ Heart Disease/Attack   ❑ Heart Pacemaker   ❑ Rheumatic Fever

(continued)

❑ Angina Pectoris   ❑ Congenital Heart Disease   ❑ Artificial Joint

❑ High Blood Pressure   ❑ Artificial Heart Valve   ❑ Weight Control Drugs (Fen-phen, Redux, Pondimin, etc.)

❑ Stroke   ❑ Heart Murmur

19. Please check any of the following that you *have had* or *have* at present:

❑ Diabetes   ❑ Sickle Cell Disease   ❑ Hepatitis/Yellow Jaundice

❑ Leukemia   ❑ Abnormal Bleeding/ Blood Disorder   ❑ Thyroid Disease

❑ Chemotherapy   ❑ Hemophilia   ❑ HIV

❑ Radiation Treatment   ❑ Kidney Disease   ❑ AIDS

❑ Anemia   ❑ Liver Disease

20. Please check any of the following that you *have had* or *have* at present:

❑ Emphysema   ❑ Asthma   ❑ Multiple Surgeries

❑ Persistent Cough   ❑ Hay Fever   ❑ Genitourinary problems (bladder, kidney, ureter, genital)

❑ Tuberculosis   ❑ Spina Bifida   ❑ Allergies; list:_____

21. Please check any of the following that you *have had* or *have* at present:

❑ Rheumatism   ❑ Stomach Ulcers   ❑ Chemical Dependency

❑ Lupus Erythematosus   ❑ Glaucoma   ❑ Tobacco Use

❑ Arthritis   ❑ Fainting or Dizzy Spells   ❑ Sexually Transmitted Disease

❑ Back Problems   ❑ Epilepsy or Seizures   ❑ Cold Sores/Fever Blisters

❑ Osteoporosis   ❑ Eating Disorder   ❑ Mental Health Care

❑ Ulcerative Colitis

22. Do you have any disease, condition, or problem not listed?   Yes   No

If so, specify _____

23. Please check any of the following medications you are currently taking:

❑ Antibiotics   ❑ Anticoagulants (Blood Thinners)   ❑ Insulin-type drug

❑ Sulfa Drugs   ❑ Medicine for High Blood Pressure   ❑ Cortisone (Steroids)

❑ Nitroglycerin   ❑ Digitalis/Drugs for Heart Trouble   ❑ Antihistamine

❑ Tranquilizers
❑ Antidepressant   ❑ Vitamins, Supplements, and/or Herbs   ❑ Dilantin/Phenobarbital (Anticonvulsants)

❑ Non-aspirin pain relievers   ❑ Hormones (Birth Control or Replacement Therapy)   ❑ Aspirin
Other: Specify_____

24. Please check any of the following that you are allergic to or have adversely reacted to:

❑ Local Anesthetics   ❑ Aspirin

❑ Penicillin/Other Antibiotics   ❑ Codeine/Other Narcotics

❑ Nitrous Oxide–Oxygen Analgesia (Gas)   Other: Specify_____

25. Do you have a latex allergy diagnosed by a doctor?   Yes   No

(continued)

To the best of my knowledge, all of the preceding answers are true and correct, and I acknowledge that my questions, if any, about inquiries set forth above have been answered to my satisfaction. I will not hold my dentist, or any other member of his or her staff, responsible for any action they take or do not take because of errors or omissions that I may have made in the completion of this form.

If I have any change in my health, or if my medicines change, I will inform the clinician at the next appointment.

_____   _____

Date   Signature of Patient, Parent, or Guardian

	DATE	BP	RESP. RATE	PULSE	PATIENT SIGNATURE	CLINICIAN SIGNATURE
1					N/A	
	DATE	BP	RESP. RATE	PULSE	PATIENT SIGNATURE	CLINICIAN SIGNATURE

Updates_____

Antibiotic Prophylaxis (reason, dosage, time)_____

Update 2

ASA and Blood Pressure Classifications

AMERICAN SOCIETY OF ANESTHESIOLOGISTS PHYSICAL STATUS CLASSIFICATION

I. Normal healthy individual
  - Treatment modifications usually not needed
  - No abnormalities found, tolerant of stress
  - Normal blood pressure: <120 and <80

II. Patient with mild to moderate systemic disease
  - Well-controlled epilepsy, asthma, non-insulin-dependent diabetes, and thyroid disorders
  - Otherwise healthy patients with allergies, or extreme dental fears
  - Prehypertension: Adult blood pressure between 120 and 139 (systolic) or 80 and 89 (diastolic)

III. Patient with severe systemic disease that limits activity but is not incapacitating
  - Stable angina pectoris, >6 months post myocardial infarction (MI)
  - Exercise-induced asthma, chronic obstructive pulmonary disease (COPD), well controlled insulin-dependent diabetes
  - Stage 1 hypertension: Adult blood pressure between 140 and 159 systolic or 90 and 99 diastolic

IV. Patient with severe systemic disease that limits activity and is a constant threat to life
  - Myocardial infarction (MI) or cerebral vascular accident (CVA) within the last 6 months
  - Uncontrolled epilepsy, diabetes, COPD with O_2
  - Stage 2 hypertension: Adult blood pressure ≥160/100

V. Moribund patient not expected to survive 24 hours with or without an operation
  - Terminal cancer
  - End-stage renal disease, hepatic disease and infectious disease
  - End-stage disease, hepatic disease and infectious disease

Source: Physical Status Classification Information compiled from American Society of Anestheeiologists (1963)

BLOOD PRESSURE CLASSIFICATIONS[a]				DENTAL GUIDELINES[b]
	SYSTOLIC		DIASTOLIC	
Normal	<120	AND	<80	Treatment modifications usually not needed Routine management Recheck in 6 months
Prehypertension	120–139	or	80–89	Routine treatment okay Discuss guidelines with patient
Stage 1 hypertension	140–159	or	90–99	Routine treatment okay Consider sedation for complex dental or surgical procedures; refer for medical consult
Stage 2 hypertension	≥160	or	≥100	
	160–179	or	100–109	Routine treatment OK[c] Consider sedation for complex dental or surgical procedures; refer for medical consult
	180–209	or	110–119	No dental treatment without medical consultation Refer for prompt medical consult
	≥210	or	≥120	No dental treatment Refer for emergency medical treatment

[a]Adapted from U.S Department of Health and Human Services, National Institutes of Health; National Heart, Lung, and Blood Institute; National High Blood Pressure Education Program (2004).
[b]Dental guidelines from Herman and Konzelman (2004)
[c]If patient has medical risk factors, such as prior myocardial infarction, angina, high coronary disease risk, prior stroke, diabetes, or kidney disease, medical consultation should be obtained before performing dental treatment.

General Rules for Cardiac Patients

1. If in doubt, obtain a medical consult from patient's physician.
2. Premedicate with sedative if fearful or apprehensive.
3. Keep appointments short, when patient is well rested, and at least 1 hour after eating. Morning appointments are best (except in congestive heart disease).
4. Verify medications.
5. Relative contraindication to vasopressors.
   Limit the amount of *epinephrine* to 0.04 mg (2.2 carpules of 1:100,000 epinephrine or 4.4 carpules of 1:200,000 epinephrine).
   Limit amount of *levonordefrin* to 0.2 mg (2.2 carpules of mepivicaine 1:20,000).
6. Do not use gingival retraction cord containing epinephrine.
7. Do not administer intraligamentary injections.
8. Use good technique to diminish stress and control pain.
9. Clinicians should be familiar with the newest American Heart Association guidelines for antibiotic premedication.

Summary Charts from CD-ROM

The information provided in the following Section III tables and charts is compiled from assorted references (See Reference List). Key references include: Malamed (2004), Little (2002), ADA Guide to Dental Therapeutics (2003), Aubertin (2004), Bennett (1984), Malamed (2000), Naftalin and Yagiela (2002), and Budenz (2002).

TABLE 1: HEATH HISTORY QUESTIONS REGARDING CARDIOVASCULAR DISEASES

In addition to the question, "Have you ever had any of the following heart conditions?" common patient history questions that could be indicators of atypical heart function may include the following:

QUESTION	POSSIBLE RISKS	SIGNIFICANCE
Medical History Question 5: Do you have chest pain upon exertion?	• Angina pectoris: chest pain caused by temporary lack of blood to the myocardium • Etiology—large meals coupled with stress or exertion	• Limit the amount of vasoconstrictor[a] • Patient must bring medication to appointment • Schedule 1 h after meals
Medical History Question 5: Do you have shortness of breath after mild exercise? Medical History Question 6: Do your ankles often swell? Medical History Question 7: Must you use multiple pillows for sleeping?	• Congestive heart failure (CHF)/atherosclerosis: likely have a decrease in blood flow through the liver that would prolong the metabolism of drugs • Likely have an increase in cardiac stroke volume leading to risk of overdose reaction • Less able to handle stress	• Limit the amount of vasoconstrictor • Use of nitrous oxide or light sedative to reduce stress • Short appointments, later in the day • Semisupine position
Medical History Question 18: Have you had repeated heart attacks or one within the last 6 mo?	• Another attack likely to occur	• Delay treatment a minimum of 6 mo • When treatment resumes, limit the amount of vasoconstrictor
Medical History Question 18: Have you had rheumatic fever, heart murmur or other congenital heart problems?	• May need pretreatment antibiotic prophylaxis • More in depth evaluation needed and possible medical consultation	• With the exception of the periodontal ligament injection, the administration of local anesthetic does *not* require antibiotic therapy; that is determined by the dental procedure to be performed • May need to limit the amount of vasoconstrictor

(continued)

QUESTION	POSSIBLE RISKS	SIGNIFICANCE
Medical History Question 18: Do you have a pacemaker?	• No known risk	• Do not use EDA or TENS equipment
Medical History Question 18: Have you had heart surgery?	• May need pretreatment antibiotic prophylaxis • More in-depth evaluation needed and possible medical consultation	• Limit the amount of vasoconstrictor
Medical History Question 18: Do you have hypertension or have you had a stroke?	• More in-depth evaluation needed and possible medical consultation	• Limit the amount of vasoconstrictor • Good aspiration *critical*
Medical History Question 23: Are you taking anticoagulants?	• Avoid deep injections when possible (e.g., PSA, inferior alveolar)	• Evaluate the procedure for excessive bleeding • May need to increase dosage prior to treatment

aWhen indicated, vasoconstrictor should be limited to 0.04 mg of epinephrine or 0.2 mg of levonordefrin.

TABLE 2: HEALTH HISTORY QUESTIONS REGARDING THYROID GLAND DYSFUNCTION

QUESTION	POSSIBLE RISKS	SIGNIFICANCE
Medical History Question 19: Do you have a hyperactive thyroid gland (hyperthyroidism) or unexplained weight loss? Additional questions that could be asked to help determine hyperthyroid condition: 1. Do you commonly experience a rapid throbbing pulse or heart rate? 2. Do you experience tremors of your arms or legs? 3. Are you very sensitive to heat and do you sweat easily? 4. Do you experience unexplained nervousness?	• Patients are reactive to catecholamines • May be sensitive to certain drugs • May be predisposed to angina and other heart diseases • May be predisposed to high blood pressure • Exaggeration of all functions	• Limit epinephrine and levonordefrin • Medical consult is advised • Thoroughly evaluate drug therapies • Liver function is generally diminished • May need to premedicate for stress if patient is anxious • Do not use epinephrine impregnated retraction cord • Do not administer a PDL injection
Do you have an underactive thyroid gland (hypothyroidism) or unexplained weight gain?	• If left untreated, may develop heart disease • Metabolism is significantly diminished	• Keep all drugs to a minimum • Normal drug doses, including anesthetic agents, can produce overdose proportions

TABLE 3: HEALTH HISTORY QUESTIONS REGARDING METABOLIC DEFICIENCIES, BLOOD DISORDERS, AND CONVULSIVE DISORDERS

QUESTION	POSSIBLE RISKS	SIGNIFICANCE
Medical History Question 19: Do you have diabetes?	• Healing may be prolonged	• Limit the amount of vasoconstrictor
Medical History Question 11: Are you thirsty much of the time? Medical History Question 12: Is your mouth frequently dry? Medical History Question 10: Do you urinate more than six times a day?	• May have correlated cardiac problems • May develop eye disorders • Frequently experience increased toxemia in pregnancy	• Dental treatment must not interfere with meals • Antibiotic premedication may be needed if there is a risk of postoperative infection • Have sugar drinks available
Not on Health History Form: Do you know if you have any type of cholinesterase deficiency? (because it is hereditary, patients usually know)	• Hydrolysis of ester anesthetic agents and may be slowed significantly	• Be cautious with amount of ester type of topical agents used • Predisposes patient to risk of overdose • Greater threat is during general anesthesia with succinylcholine use
Medical History Question 19: Have you had jaundice, hepatitis A or B, blood diseases such as hemophilia? Medical History Question 21: Do you have a chemical dependency to drugs or alcohol? Medical History Question 19: Are you aware of liver damage?	• The half-life of amide local anesthetics may be significantly prolonged • Risk of infection via blood or saliva is increased	• Limit the amount of amide anesthetic • Low tolerance to any drugs • Limit any type of medication including esters or pretreatment sedative • Predisposes patient to risk of overdose
Medical History Question 19: Are you aware of any kidney damage or disease you might have?	• A portion of all anesthetic agents and vasoconstrictors reach the kidneys unmetabolized	• Limit the amount of agents administered • Predisposes patient to risk of overdose • Antibiotic premedication may be needed • Low tolerance to any drugs
Medical History Question 21: Do you have epilepsy or experience other types of seizures?	• Stress reduction protocol should be used	• Use vasoconstrictor if possible • Depends on medications patient may be taking

Note: Seek medical consultation if in doubt about any of the above conditions.

Summary of Contraindications for Local Anesthetics and Vasoconstrictors

SUMMARY OF CONTRAINDICATIONS FOR LOCAL ANESTHETICS

Absolute Contraindication

1. Documented allergy to local anesthetic drug. Do not use anesthetics from same chemical group.

Relative Contraindications

ASSOCIATED DISEASE	SIGNIFICANCE
1. Malignant hyperthermia	Use amides judiciously
2. Atypical pseudo-cholinesterase	Do not use esters; use amides
3. Significant liver dysfunction	Use esters or amides, but use judiciously
4. Renal dysfunction	Use esters or amides, but use judiciously
5. Methemoglobinemia	Use amide, but do not use prilocaine
6. Patients taking acetaminophen or phenacetin	Long-term basis may cause methemoglobinemia; use amide but avoid use of prilocaine
7. Significant cardiovascular disease Patients taking digoxin (Lanoxin), enalapril (Vasotec), furosemide (Lasix)	Limit amount of vasoconstrictor; use anesthetic with no or low concentration of vasoconstrictor, e.g., 3% mepivacaine, 4% prilocaine plain, 4% prilocaine with 1:200,000 epinephrine, 0.5% bupivacaine with 1:200,000 epinephrine, 4% articaine with 1:200,000 epinephrine
8. Clinical hyperthyroidism	Same as above for cardiovascular disease
9. Patients taking cimetadine (Tagamet, Zantac) on a regular basis	Drug reduces capacity of liver to metabolize amides; reduce dosage by one half
10. Antianxiety drugs: benzodiazepines, e.g., diazepam (Valium)	Minimize dosages of all anesthetics

SUMMARY OF CONTRAINDICATIONS FOR VASOCONSTRICTORS

Absolute Contraindications

1. Recent myocardial infarction (3 to 6 months)
2. Recent coronary bypass surgery (3 to 6 months)
3. Uncontrolled high blood pressure
4. Daily angina or uncontrolled arrhythmias
5. Sulfite allergies (especially in patients with steroid-dependent asthma)
6. Uncontrolled diabetes (causes hyperglycemic effect)
7. Pheochromocytoma—catecholamine-producing tumors
8. Uncontrolled hyperthyroidism

Relative Contraindications

Note: For the following, limit amount of epinephrine to 0.04 mg; limit amount of levonordefrin to 0.2 mg per appointment.

ASSOCIATED DISEASE	SIGNIFICANCE
1. Patients taking tricyclic antidepressants, e.g., amitriptyline with perphenazine (Triavil), Elavil, desipramine hydrochloride (Norpramin), Tofranil, trimipramine (Aventyl), protrityline (Vivactil), etc.	Increases effects of epinephrine; levonordefrin should be avoided; both may cause acute hypertension and cardiac dysrhythmia
2. Patient taking phenothiazides, e.g., acetophenazine (Tindal), chlorpromazine (Thorazine), perphenazine (Trilafon), triflupromazine (Vesprin), thioridazine (Mellaril), etc.	Increased risk of hypotension; epinephrine stimulates beta receptors; combined with drug creates unbalance in body
3. Patient taking nonselective beta blockers, e.g., propranolol (Inderal), Corgard, Blocadren	Increased hypertension resulting in rebound bradycardia; potential cardiac arrest; if hemostasis is not essential, consider using local anesthetic without vasopressor
4. Cocaine abusers	Avoid use of vasopressors; may lead to myocardial infarction Because of the prevalence of cocaine use in certain population groups, clinicans should be aware of the seriousness of using vasopressors with patients using this drug. Cocaine stimulates norepinephrine release and inhibits its reuptake. It can cause tachycardia and dysrhythmias, which in turn increase cardiac output and oxygen requirements. If ischemia occurs, potentially lethal dysrhythmias, anginal pain, myocardial infarction, or cardiac arrest may result. If possible, vasopressors should not be administered when cocaine is in the system. Clinicians should *never* use epinephrine-impregnated gingival retraction cord with these patients.
5. Glaucoma	Limit amount of vasopressor; causes increased ocular pressure
6. Controlled diabetes	Vasoconstrictors directly oppose effect of insulin, possible changes in blood levels of glucose
7. Controlled hyperthyroidism	Vasoconstrictor effect increased
8. Controlled high blood pressure	Very controversial; risks associated with vasoconstrictors—increase in blood pressure

Complications

I. COMPLICATIONS ATTRIBUTED TO SOLUTION USED

COMPLICATION	CAUSE	SYMPTOMS	TREATMENT	PREVENTION
Toxicity	Inadvertent IV injection; Too large a volume; Slow biotransformation; Slow elimination; Unusually rapid absorption	Stimulation, i.e., high blood pressure (BP), pulse, and respiration; patient becomes talkative, apprehensive, excited, followed by depression, i.e., low BP, pulse, respiration; convulsions, unconsciousness; death due to respiratory depression	Discontinue treatment; Position patient; Maintain airway and provide supplemental oxygen. **Summon emergency personnel.** Monitor vital signs; Provide basic life support	Aspirate; Use smallest possible volume of the drug. Use weakest concentration possible; Inject slowly; Use vasoconstrictor, when possible Thorough patient evaluation
Allergic reaction	A specific antigen-antibody reaction	Rash, urticaria, edema, wheezing, dyspnea, flushing, mucous membrane congestion	Antihistamines, e.g., diphenhydramine hydrochloride (Benadryl) Oxygen	Thorough medical history
Anaphylactoid reaction	Form of allergy	Suddenness of onset, complete collapse; loss of consciousness; imperceptible pulse and respiration; cyanotic or ashen gray color	Prompt action **Summon emergency personnel;** Administer treatment as needed; Basic life support; Administer epinephrine	Thorough medical history
Idiosyncrasy (any reaction that cannot be classified as toxic or allergic)	Usually considered a genetic deviation or aberration; aberration remains undetected until a specific drug creates its bizarre clinical manifestation	Vary; impossible to outline in advance (may also be psychogenic)	Symptomatic: basic life support	Unable to ascertain in advance Obtain thorough health history; do not expose patient to anything related to a past reaction
Local reactions caused by anesthetic solution	Contaminated solutions (this is rare because of manufacturers' high standards of asepsis)	Local tissue irritation or burning	None	Check cartridge for debris; Buy anesthetic from reliable manufacturer; Inject slowly

(continued)

COMPLICATION	CAUSE	SYMPTOMS	TREATMENT	PREVENTION
Sloughing of tissue	Topical anesthetic for prolonged period of time; secondary to use of vasoconstrictors	Epithelial desquamation Apthous ulcer	Reassure patient	Use topical anesthetics properly Use low concentrations of vasoconstrictors
Edema	Could be: trauma during injection; infection; allergy; hemorrhage; injecting contaminated solution	Pain Dysfunction in region May lead to compromised airway (tongue, larynx, pharynx)	Decrease swelling quickly May need analgesics or antihistamines	Good technique; Aseptic technique; Thorough medical history
Lip/soft tissue injury	Inadvertently biting oneself while anesthetized; most common in children or mentally and physically challenged patients.	Trauma Pain Swelling	Analgesics for pain Warm saline rinses Keep lubricated	Warn patients, parents/ guardians Good communication Use short-acting anesthetic if possible.

II. COMPLICATIONS ATTRIBUTED TO NEEDLE INSERTION OR TECHNICAL COMPLICATIONS

COMPLICATION	CAUSE	SYMPTOMS	TREATMENT	PREVENTION
Fainting	Form of shock— sometimes due to seeing the needle	Low BP, pallor, coolness of skin, perspiration, light-headedness, nausea	Lower chair so legs are elevated Have ammonia ampoule handy	Keep patient as calm as possible Keep needle out of view
Muscle trismus	Trauma to muscle during needle insertion; also irritating solution, hemorrhage or low-grade infection Multiple needle penetrations	Muscle soreness Limited movement of mandible	Heat therapy (20 min/h) Analgesics—ibuprofen Physiotherapy—gum chewing Warm saline rinses— 1 tsp in 12 oz water; time (48–72 h)	Watch landmarks Good technique Aseptic technique Avoid repeated needle insertion. Limit number of injections in same area
Pain (hyperesthesia)	Poor technique Rapid deposition of solution Needle with barbs	Pain	Reassure patient	Use topical Use sharp needles change every three to four injections. Good technique
Infection	Nonsterile instruments, etc. Improper technique.	Low-grade inflammation which may result in trismus	If persistent, penicillin or erythromycin	Aseptic technique

(continued)

COMPLICATION	CAUSE	SYMPTOMS	TREATMENT	PREVENTION
Broken needle	Primary cause is patient making a sudden unanticipated movement; needles of smaller gauge are more likely to break; needles previously bent are more likely to break		Instruct patient not to move; keep hand in patient's mouth; if fragment protruding, remove with cotton pliers or hemostat. If fragment is lost, refer to oral surgeon for consult	Do not force needle against resistance. Do not attempt to change direction of needle while embedded in tissue (withdraw slightly) Use disposable needles Know landmarks Do not insert needle so far that it is out of view
Hematoma	Torn blood vessel Improper technique	Swelling; discoloration Possible soreness and limitation of movement	Direct pressure for 10 min; Ice pack; heat after 4–6 h (20 min/h) Gradually resorbs in 7–14 days	Use good technique Can occur even with proper technique
Paresthesia	Trauma to nerve Contaminated solutions resulting in edema Hemorrhage into or around nerve fiber	Persistent anesthesia for many hours or days.	Examine and reassure patient Usually resolves within 8 weeks Consult oral surgeon if not resolved within 1 year	Use good technique Aseptic technique Do not store carpules in disinfecting solution Minimize number of injections in same area
Facial nerve paralysis	Injecting anesthetic into parotid gland capsule	Loss of motor function to muscles of facial expression; transitory Dehydration of cornea	Wait for anesthesia to wear off; manually close eyes periodically; reassure patient	Good technique with inferior alveolar injection
Postanesthetic intraoral lesions	Trauma to oral tissues	Recurrent apthous stomatitis Herpes simplex	Treat symptom	No prevention
Burning	Rapid injection pH of solution low Warm solution Contaminated solution	May cause trismus, edema, or paresthesia	No particular treatment—manage given situation	Inject slowly Local anesthetic with vasoconstrictor has lower pH Warmer solutions may feel "hot" to patient Sterile technique—no contaminated solution

Emergency Reference Chart

EMERGENCY	SIGNS/SYMPTOMS	PROCEDURE
Hyperventilation syndrome	Light-headedness, giddiness, anxiety, confusion, dizziness Overbreathing/feelings of suffocation Deep respiration/palpitations and tingling or numbness	Terminate oral procedure Remove objects from mouth Position for comfortable breathing Loosen tight collar and reassure patient Ask patient to breath deeply into a paper bag
Syncope	Pale gray face, anxiety, dilated pupils, weakness, giddiness, dizziness, faintness Nausea, profuse perspiration, rapid pulse first, followed by slow, shallow breathing, drop in BP and loss of consciousness	Position: Trendelenburg and loosen tight collar and belt, cold damp towel on forehead; crush ammonia under patients nose; keep warm and monitor vitals; keep airway open, require O_2 in supine position for 10 min after recovery
Angina	Sudden crushing pain in substernal area, pain may radiate to shoulder, neck, and arms; pallor, faintness, shallow breathing, anxiety, fear	Position: Upright for comfortable breathing, nitro sublingually 1 tablet every 5 min, no more than 3 Administer O_2 if needed and reassure patient
Myocardial infarction	Sudden pain similar to angina pectoris, which also may radiate, but lasts longer; pallor, cold and clammy skin, cyanosis; nausea, breathing difficulty, marked weakness, anxiety and fear; may lose consciousness	Position: Head up for comfort breathing; monitor vitals, administer O_2 if needed; nitrous oxide 25% to alleviate anxiety; reassure patient; call for medical assistance, transfer to supine position, begin basic life support (BLS), cardiopulmonary resuscitation
Stroke	Dizziness, vertigo, and transient paresthesia or weakness on one side; transient speech defects	Turn patient toward affected side; semiupright, loosen collar, and reassure patient; monitor vitals, do not give sedative, stimulant, or narcotic; clear airway and seek medical assistance; use O_2 only if patient is having respiratory problems
Hypoglycemia	Sudden onset; skin is moist, cold, pale; confused, nervous, anxious, pounding pulse, salivation, normal to shallow respiration; if continues, convulsion possible, loss of consciousness	Conscious patient oral sugar, observe for 1 h; determine time since previous meal, arrange appointment following food intake; unconscious patient BLS; supine, maintain airway, administer O_2 **Summon emergency personnel**

(continued)

EMERGENCY	SIGNS/SYMPTOMS	PROCEDURE
Diabetic coma	Slow onset; skin is flush and dry; breath has fruity odor; dry mouth; low BP; weak rapid pulse, exaggerated respiration; coma	Conscious patient terminate oral procedure; obtain medical care, keep patient warm; unconscious patient BLS; urgent medical assistance **Summon emergency personnel**
Epileptic seizures	Anxiety and depression; pale, may become cyanotic; muscular contractions; loss of consciousness	Supine, protect patient from injury; do not force anything into mouth, open airway, monitor vitals; allow patient to sleep during postconvulsive phase
Status epilepticus		If lasts longer than 5 min, **summon emergency personnel,** administer anticonvulsant, e.g., diazepam IV
Allergic reaction	Red, itching skin, localized mucous membrane swelling, wheezing, dyspnea, possible obstruction from swelling, respiratory distress	Give antihistamine, position upright, give O$_2$, maintain airway, get medical assistance; administer IV epinephrine if very severe
Anesthetic overdose	Anxious, restless, confused, apprehensive; rapid pulse and breathing, then to a depressive phase—BP lowers, respiration decreases, tremors, seizures	Stop injection, position supine, loosen clothing, reassure patient, monitor vitals, give O$_2$, get medical assistance, may require BLS; **summon emergency personnel** if continues; give diazapam if seizures last longer than 5 min
Vasoconstrictor overdose or sensitivity	Pallor, dizziness, throbbing headache, anxiety, tremors, heart palpitations, elevated BP, elevated heart rate; if severe, possible myocardial infarction	Terminate procedure, sit up erect, reassure patient, monitor vital signs; administer O$_2$, BLS, **summon emergency personnel** if continues

SECTION III LEARNING ACTIVITIES

DIRECTIONS: Read through the following patient scenarios and, based on the information provided, select an appropriate anesthetic for each of the cases.

SELECTION OF LOCAL ANESTHETIC AGENTS FOR PATIENTS WITH COMPROMISED HEALTH HISTORIES

1. A 35-year-old woman patient who is taking a tricyclic antidepressant is scheduled for a 1-hour appointment. You plan to scale the maxillary right quadrant today. What anesthetic(s) should you avoid?
2. A 5-year-old boy who weighs 55 lb is moving out of town soon so his mother does not want to delay treatment. Restorative treatment on two quadrants is scheduled for completion today. There are no significant findings on the child's medical history. What anesthetic would you use? Provide rationale for your selection.
3. A 45-year-old 110-lb woman is scheduled to have a crown prep today on tooth #30. Her medical history indicates she has hyperthyroidism and is taking appropriate medication for her condition. What anesthetic would you use? What is the maximum recommended amount of the anesthetic you could use for this patient during this appointment?
4. A 60-year-old man is scheduled to have two amalgam restorations placed on the maxillary left quadrant. He reports on his medical history that he is taking the drug Inderal to control his high blood pressure. What anesthetic would be appropriate for this 1-hour appointment?
5. A 70-year-old woman is scheduled for a 4-month recall cleaning appointment. Her mandibular anterior teeth are very sensitive. On her updated medical history she states that she has been diagnosed with glaucoma since her last dental appointment. What injections would you give to anesthetize these mandibular anterior teeth? What anesthetic would be appropriate for use?

COMPLICATIONS ATTRIBUTED TO NEEDLE INSERTION

1. You have just given a right mandibular inferior alveolar injection. Your patient states that the "whole side of his face feels numb" and he cannot close his eye on that side. Refer to the picture below of this patient's face. What is the most likely cause of these symptoms?

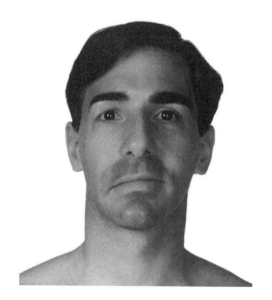

2. The patient in your chair is a 20-year-old man who has an appointment for a small restoration on tooth #5. There are no significant findings on his medical history. You have just given him ⅔ cartridge of mepivacaine 3% for an infiltration injection over that tooth. He becomes pale, his pupils dilate, and he begins to perspire. What do these signs indicate may be happening? What should you do to manage this situation?

3. You have just given your patient a left PSA injection using lidocaine 2% 1:100,000 epineph-rine. Immediately you notice swelling and slight discoloration of the left cheek. What is the most likely cause of this swelling? What steps should you take to manage this complication?

COMPLICATIONS ATTRIBUTED TO THE SOLUTION ADMINISTERED (SYSTEMIC)

1. A young boy who was treated in the office yesterday for composite restorations on teeth I and J returns today, due to pain on the underside of his lip. One carpule of 2% lidocaine 1:100,000 epinephrine was used for his infiltration injections. Referring to the picture of the boy's lip, what is the most likely cause of this lesion?

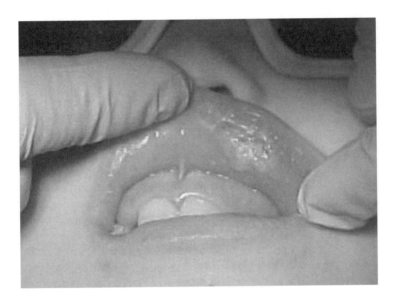

2. Your patient needs a mesio-occluso-distal (MOD) restoration on tooth #19. He has asthma and takes prescribed steroid medication for that condition. You give him 1 carpule of Articaine 1:100,000 for the left inferior alveolar (IA) injection. Immediately he begins to get a rash on his chest. Within a few minutes you notice red wheals/urticaria on his left arm. He says he feels like he is having difficulty breathing. What do you think may be causing these symptoms? What should you do to manage this complication?

3. You have just administered an infraorbital injection on a 30-year-old woman whose health his-tory is within normal limits. She states that while you were depositing the anesthetic she felt a strong burning sensation throughout the entire injection, worse at the beginning of the injec-tion and lessening slightly toward the end. You used ⅔ cartridge of 3% plain mepivacaine. What are possible causes of this sensation? What should you tell your patient?

4. Conduct an evidence-based review of the most current contraindications for administering local anesthetic agents and/or their vasoconstrictors. Identify any changes that have been reported since the publication of this CD.

ANSWER KEY FOR SECTION III ACTIVITIES

SELECTION OF LOCAL ANESTHETIC AGENTS FOR PATIENTS WITH COMPROMISED HEALTH HISTORIES

1. Vasoconstrictors are relative contraindications for patients taking tricyclic antidepressants. Use of vasoconstrictors could potentially cause acute hypertension and cardiac dysrhythmia. If using an anesthetic with epinephrine, the amount of epinephrine should be kept to a minimum (0.04 mg). Therefore, if using an anesthetic with 1:100,000 epinephrine or 1:20,000 levonordefrin, no more than 2 cartridges should be used. If using an anesthetic with 1:200,000 epinephrine, no more than 4 cartridges should be administered.

2. The young boy's medical history is within normal limits; therefore, no local anesthetic is contraindicated. However, the prudent clinician must be sure to calculate the maximum recommended dosage for the patient weighing 55 lb. The local anesthetic will be the limiting agent. If using the following anesthetics, the maximum number of carpules is calculated:
   2% lidocaine   55 lbs × 2 mg/lb = 110 mg max
       36 mg lidocaine per carpule
       110/36 = 3 carpules
   3% mepivacaine   55 × 2 mg/lb = 110 mg max
       54 mg mepivacaine per carpule
       110/54 = 2 carpules
   4% prilocaine   55 × 2.7 mg/lb = 148 mg max
       72 mg prilocaine per carpule
       148/72 = 2 carpules
   With two entire quadrants scheduled for today's appointment, it would be wise to assume you may need to use more than 2 carpules. As such, lidocaine would be the most appropriate anesthetic of the three listed above for today's appointment. An anesthetic that should be avoided for a child of this age is bupivacaine (Marcaine). It provides too long a duration of soft tissue anesthesia, and the child would be prone to post-treatment injury of the tissues.

3. Vasoconstrictors are a relative contraindication for patients with hyperthyroidism. This patient is on medication and controlled; however, to minimize risk it is always prudent to err on the side of caution and stay within the recommended dosages for a relative contraindication. For hyperthyroidism those maximum recommended dosages are 0.04 mg epinephrine and 0.2 mg levonordefrin. Therefore, if you use an anesthetic with 1:100,000 epinephrine, no more than 2 carpules should be used. Likewise, no more than 4 carpules of 1:200,000 epinephrine should be used, or no more than 2 carpules of 1:20,000 levonordefrin. This patient weighs only 110 lb; however, because she has hyperthyroidism, the limiting agent will be the vasoconstrictor, which is not weight dependent. As such, the calculation for her weight is not an issue for the amount of anesthetic given.

4. This 60-year-old man is taking a nonselective beta blocker to control his high blood pressure. Vasoconstrictors should be used with extreme caution for patients on these types of medications. As in scenario 3 above, limit the amount of vasoconstrictor: for 1:100,0000 epinephrine, limit amount to no more than 2 carpules; for 1:200,000 epinephrine no more than 4 carpules; for 1:20,000 levonordefrin, limit amount to 2 carpules. Any of the anesthetics available could be used for this procedure as long as the clinician adheres to these limits. To minimize risk, give 1 carpule of anesthetic very slowly and monitor closely prior to giving another dosage.

5. For this 4-month recall appointment you would most likely want to finish all of her teeth in one appointment. Bilateral mandibular blocks are *rarely* indicated, due to the possibility of soft tissue injury. Therefore, a more appropriate treatment plan would be to administer bilateral incisive injections, which would anesthetize all the mandibular anterior teeth without the

extensive soft tissue anesthesia. Glaucoma is a relative contraindication to the use of vasocon-strictors due to the possibility of increased ocular pressure caused by the use of vasoconstric-tors. Therefore, you would follow the same guidelines as stated in scenarios 3 and 4 above for the other relative contraindications and their maximum recommended dosages of vasocon-strictors. Again, the guidelines are as follows: 1:100,0000 epinephrine, limit amount to no more than 2 carpules; 1:200,000 epinephrine, no more than 4 carpules; 1:20,000 levonorde-frin, limit amount to 2 carpules.

COMPLICATIONS ATTRIBUTED TO NEEDLE INSERTION

1. This patient is most likely experiencing facial nerve paralysis. This temporary paralysis can occur when the facial nerve, which runs through the parotid gland, is anesthetized during the inferior alveolar injection. If bone is not contacted when giving an inferior alveolar injection, and the solution is injected too posteriorly into the parotid gland, the facial nerve can be anes-thetized and cause the signs demonstrated on the picture.
2. The signs this patient is demonstrating indicate syncope. To manage this emergency, you should place the patient in a supine position, explain what is happening, and try to alleviate his anxiety. If symptoms do not dissipate, pass an ammonia carpule below the nostrils and have patient breathe. Usually this emergency resolves quickly. Reassure the patient and perform scheduled treatment if patient is comfortable and wants to continue with the appointment.
3. The most likely cause of the symptoms described in this scenario is the development of a hematoma from the accidental "nick" of a blood vessel in the pterygoid plexus. Because of the close proximity of the pterygoid plexus to the PSA branches, this is not an uncommon com-plication during this injection. You should immediately place ice on the cheek and have the patient hold with pressure on this area. Explain to the patient what occurred and recommend heat compresses with warm moist towels every 20 min after 4 to 6 h or beginning the next day. Explain there may be some minor soreness and discomfort in the area and that bruising and discoloration will last 10 to 14 days. Make certain to inform the patient that no permanent injury will result from this occurrence.

COMPLICATIONS ATTRIBUTED TO THE SOLUTION (SYSTEMIC)

1. From the appearance of the lesion on the lip, the child most likely chewed on his lip while it was still anesthetized after treatment was completed. To avoid this fairly common and painful complication, it is imperative to explain to the adult who chaperones the child of the need to carefully monitor a child who is still numb. Inform the adult that the numbness may last for several hours, and lip biting during that time period will undoubtedly lead to postanesthetic complications.
2. This patient's symptoms are indicative of an allergic reaction. The steps you should take include the following: give the patient an antihistamine, monitor to see if symptoms begin to resolve, and check for breathing difficulty. If symptoms worsen, paramedics should be called, the patient monitored, and progressive steps taken as needed. It is possible that this reaction occurred due to the sodium bisulfites (used as a preservative for the vasoconstrictor) contained in the local anesthetic cartridge. Patients with asthma taking steroid medications are at a sig-nificant risk for allergic reaction to sodium bisulfites.
3. If the anesthetic has a vasoconstrictor, it is possible to attribute a burning sensation to the lower pH of these anesthetics. However, because this anesthetic does not contain a vasocon-strictor, there must be another explanation. You look over at the local anesthetic container and notice someone has put a 4 × 4 gauze square saturated in alcohol over the top of the carpules. It is likely this alcohol was absorbed through the rubber diaphragm and a small amount deposited in the solution. Contamination of an anesthetic agent with alcohol would likely cause a burning sensation while injecting the solution.

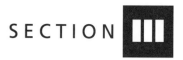
Potential Complications/ Quizzes

Physical Evaluation

1. What is the dental treatment consideration for a patient with a blood pressure reading of 180 over 110?
   a. Provide routine dental treatment and recheck in 6 months
   b. Recheck and if still elevated, recommend patient seek emergency care.
   c. Recheck and if still this high implement stress reduction protocol and deliver routine dental treatment
   d. Recheck and if still this high seek medical consultation prior to treatment.

2. How many premature ventricular contractions per minute may indicate a patient should seek medical consultation?
   a. One
   b. Two
   c. Three
   d. Four
   e. Five

3. The normal heart rate is approximately how many beats per minute?
   a. 16 to 18
   b. 50 to 75
   c. 60 to 100
   d. 75 to 125
   e. 125 to 150

4. What is the maximum amount of epinephrine a patient with a history of cardiovascular disease should receive per appointment?
   a. 0.01 mg
   b. 0.02 mg
   c. 0.04 mg
   d. 0.2 mg
   e. 1 mg

5. If a patient has had a heart attack, how long should elective dental treatment be delayed?
   a. 2 months
   b. 3 months
   c. 6 months
   d. 1 year
   e. Patient may have elective treatment if on medication and no current problems

6. Pretreatment antibiotics are absolutely indicated if a patient has had rheumatic fever.
   a. True
   b. False

7. A patient with asthma who is taking steroid medications should not be given which of the following?
   a. Epinephrine
   b. Levonordefrin
   c. Lidocaine 1:100,000
   d. Sodium bisulfites
   e. All of the above

8. What is the treatment protocol if a patient has controlled hyperthyroidism?
   a. You should not use epinephrine
   b. You should not use any vasoconstrictor
   c. You should limit the amount of vasoconstrictor
   d. You should decrease the amount of local anesthetic agent to half of the recommended dose
   e. a and b

9. Vasoconstrictors should be used in limited amounts for which of the following conditions?
   a. Hepatitis
   b. Diabetes
   c. Liver disease
   d. Patient with atypical pseudocholinesterase
   e. b and c

10. Methemoglobinemia is a condition characterized by what type of dysfunction in the body?
    a. Congenital
    b. Hereditary
    c. Acquired
    d. a and b
    e. May be any of the above

11. Which anesthetics should not be used if a patient has a history of methemoglobinemia?
    a. Prilocaine
    b. Benzocaine
    c. Articaine
    d. a and b
    e. a and c

12. Amides should be used in limited amounts in patients with what condition?
    a. Liver dysfunction
    b. Patient taking any type of ulcer medication
    c. Patient with pseudocholinesterase
    d. Patient with diabetes
    e. All of the above

Potential Complications

1. Muscle trismus is an example of a primary complication; it is also transient.
   a. The first part of the statement is true; the second part is false
   b. The first part of the statement is false; the second part is true
   c. Both parts of the statement are true
   d. Both parts of the statement are false

2. Muscle trismus can be avoided by:
   a. Not injecting into a blood vessel
   b. Avoiding repeated insertions of the needle
   c. Allowing the patient to get up and walk around briefly
   d. Placing the patient in a supine position
   e. All of the above

3. The recommended treatment for hematomas is:
   a. Ignore it and it will go away
   b. Get the patient out of the office before he discovers it
   c. Inform the patient of its presence
   d. Recommend hot packs for the next few days
   e. Recommend cold packs for the next few days
   f. Recommend cold packs for the first 24 hours, then hot packs, as needed
   g. c and d only
   h. c and f only

4. Overzealous application of some topical anesthetics can cause:
   a. Muscle trismus
   b. Tissue sloughing
   c. Hematomas
   d. Edema
   e. Transient paralysis

5. The *first* step in the management of simple syncope is:
   a. Place a cold pack on the patient's forehead
   b. Assure that the patient in a supine position
   c. Administer vasopressor drugs
   d. Administer oxygen
   e. Pass ammonia ampoule under the nose

6. Which of the following is an example of a secondary, transient complication?
   a. Hematoma
   b. Burning on injection
   c. Pain on withdrawal of the needle
   d. Long-term paresthesia
   e. Broken needle during the injection

7. A patient who has a reaction of wheals and respiratory distress, 5 min after you administer local anesthesia, is most likely suffering from what condition?
   a. Myocardial infarction
   b. Local anesthetic overdose
   c. Allergic reaction
   d. Seizure
   e. Syncope

8. To resolve the condition of the above patient, this patient may need which of the following treatments?
   a. 0.3 mg epinephrine 1:1,000
   b. Administer an antihistamine
   c. Administer oxygen
   d. Place patient in semireclined position

9. What is the most frequent cause of overdose toxicity?
   a. Patient weight
   b. Interaction with other drugs
   c. Inadvertent intravenous injection
   d. Presence of disease in patients

10. Which of the following is the single most important step in preventing an overdose from intravascular administration of local anesthetic?
   a. Use a needle no smaller than 25 gauge
   b. Aspirate in at least two planes before injection
   c. Slowly inject the local anesthetic solution
   d. Observe the patient following administration of the drug
   e. Knowing the correct anatomy of injection area

11. A reaction that cannot be explained by any known pharmacologic or biochemical mechanism is:
   a. An allergic reaction
   b. An idiosyncratic reaction
   c. Usually caused by the operator
   d. Usually caused by psychological condition
   e. b and d

12. The best prevention for preventing an idiosyncratic reaction is:
   a. Current knowledge of cardiopulmonary resuscitation
   b. A readily available current and complete emergency drug kit
   c. Fully pressurized oxygen tanks
   d. Stay away from anything that may have caused the reaction in the past

13. What are possible causes of paresthesia?
   a. Trauma to the nerve
   b. Contaminated local anesthetic solution
   c. Hemorrhage in the area of injection
   d. Any of the above

14. What can cause a burning sensation during an injection?
   a. Solution is contaminated
   b. Solution is injected into a muscle
   c. Solution contains a vasoconstrictor
   d. Solution is injected into a blood vessel
   e. a and c

15. Branches of which nerve are located in the parotid gland that can cause paralysis of the face and eye if inadvertently injected?
   a. Glossopharyngeal nerve
   b. Temporal nerve
   c. Facial nerve
   d. Infraorbital nerve
   e. Optic nerve

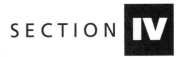
Risk Management

Summary of Characteristics of Good Communication Skills

CHARACTERISTIC	IMPORTANCE
Inform patient	Explaining to the patient in a kind, considerate approach the anticipated extent of discomfort, and informing the patient of methods available to relieve any pain indicate to the patient that his or her comfort is of prime importance. Such explanations are helpful in gaining the patient's confidence in the clinician, particularly for patients who have never had an injection before.
Show empathy, respect, and warmth	Showing respect for each individual's feelings is critical to a successful clinician–patient relationship.
Two important nonverbal behaviors:	Whether a person is speaking or listening, nonverbal behaviors are being observed and cannot be overlooked. They are crucial to effective communication.
1. Body orientation	Critical to the interpretation of a message because body language often speaks louder than our words.
2. Effective eye contact	Expresses interest and a desire to listen.
Two important verbal behaviors:	It is impossible to accurately interpret a complete message by observing only nonverbal behaviors.
1. Active listening	Requires the clinician to pay complete attention to what the patient is saying and to be responsive. It is important for the clinician to remain nonjudgmental and to concentrate on understanding what the patient is saying.
	Four principles for improving listening comprehension: 1. Anticipate where the conversation is going 2. Objectively weigh the information being presented by the patient 3. Periodically review and mentally summarize what is being said 4. Pay attention to the nonverbal behavior (Mears)
2. Paraphrasing	Can also be referred to as clarifying, reflecting, feedback, or perception check. It is a means for allowing the clinician to summarize to the patient (or vice versa) what has been heard or seen. Paraphrasing allows both parties to verify both verbal and nonverbal behaviors, allowing them to stay on course and be more involved in the discussion.

Information in the above chart was compiled primarily from Bolton (1979), David (1987), Guaza (1982) and Mears (1994).

Self-Assessment of Communication Skills

Patient Name_____   Date_____

QUESTIONS TO ASK YOURSELF	YES	NO
1. Did I show empathy, respect, and warmth while discussing the patient's needs, feelings, and expectations?		
2. Did I use body orientation and eye contact while speaking and listening to the patient?		
3. Did I actively listen to what the patient said?		
4. Did I accurately paraphrase the patient's message?		
5. Did I limit my responses to three to five sentences?		
6. Did I anticipate where the conversation was going?		
7. Did I objectively weigh information presented?		
8. Did I review and mentally summarize what was said?		
9. Did I pay attention to nonverbal behavior?		

Based on the answers to the above questions, how could I more effectively communicate with this patient:

Guide to Local Anesthesia Informed Consent and Documentation

Note: Provide comments as applicable in each area. Italicized words are sample comments.
Date_____
- **Preoperative health history evaluation discussed**
  Comments: *"My gums are sensitive and bleed when I brush"*
  Clinician: *"These are signs of periodontal (gum) disease; the local anesthesia recommended will make you more comfortable during treatment."*
- **Vital signs:** BP:_____ Pulse: _____ Resp: _____

Advantages discussed

  ❏ Comfort of patient: *"likes comfort idea"*
  ❏ Absence of pain during treatment
  ❏ Comfort of clinician to do most thorough treatment
  ❏ Time management: NA (not applicable)

- **Risks discussed**
  - ❑ Slight temporary stiffness in jaw
  - ❑ Prolonged numbness in area
  - ❑ Some swelling or bruising in area (hematoma)
  - ❑ Allergic or toxic response
  - ❑ Tissue sloughing at site
  - ❑ Intraoral lesion after injection
  - ❑ Discomfort on injection
  - ❑ Infection
  - ❑ Self-inflicted injury to lips or tongue
  - ❑ Temporary facial paralysis

  Comments: *"Wow, is it really risky?"*
  Clinician: *reaffirmed "risks minimal and extremely rare"*
- **Patient concern discussed; all questions answered**
  - ❑ No comments:
  - ❑ Comments:
- **Alternative option discussed:** Treatment without local anesthesia
  - ❑ Chance of deposits remaining greater; area: *six areas*
  - ❑ Inflammation might continue; area: *six areas*
  - ❑ Discomfort during treatment

Comments:_____

- **Preinstruction and postinstruction discussed**
  - ❑ Numbness time: *2 to 3 hours*
  - ❑ Bite cheek, lips, tongue: *2 to 3 hours*
- **Adverse reactions, complications, or side effects**
  - ❑ At time of treatment: *none*
  - ❑ After appointment by telephone: *NA*

I have been informed of the benefits and potential risks involved with local anesthesia.
  - ❑ I do consent to _____
  - ❑ I do *not* consent to _____
  - ❑ Patient or guardian signature _____

Specific Injection(s); Type and Amount of Local Anesthetic Administered

Injection administered
- ❑ Inferior alveolar
- ❑ Lingual
- ❑ Buccal
- ❑ Posterior superior alveolar
- ❑ Middle superior alveolar
- ❑ Anterior superior alveolar
- ❑ Infiltration (list tooth number) _____
- ❑ Other (list) _____

Location site
- ❑ MXL
- ❑ MXR
- ❑ MDL
- ❑ MDR

Types of anesthetic
- ❑ Lidocaine
- ❑ Prilocaine
- ❑ Mepivacaine
- ❑ Bupivacaine
- ❑ Articaine

Vasoconstrictor
- ❑ Epinephrine
- ❑ 1:50,000
- ❑ 1:100,000
- ❑ 1:200,000
- ❑ Levonordefrin
- ❑ 1:20,000

Amount of Anesthetic # cartridges____2____# milligrams ____72____.
Amount of Vasoconstrictor # milligrams___0.036____.
Clinician Signature_____

Informed Consent for Dental Hygiene Care

Following an assessment of my oral conditions and case presentation about the findings, I have been informed of the recommended plan for treatment, alternative treatment, fees for treatment, number of appointments, and the benefits and risks involved with and without treatment. The services I understand and consent to receiving include (check the box):

- ❏ Education about care for my mouth
- ❏ Instrumentation (removal of deposits)
- ❏ Stain removal (selective polishing)
- ❏ Soft tissue curettage
- ❏ Fluoride application
- ❏ Pit and fissure sealants
- ❏ Radiographs (x-rays)
- ❏ Polishing of my fillings (amalgam polishing)
- ❏ Recontouring of my fillings (overhang removal)
- ❏ Injections (anesthesia)
- ❏ Gas (nitrous oxide analgesia)

- ❏ Placement of fillings (restorations)
- ❏ Impressions for study models or athletic mouthguards
- ❏ Subgingival irrigation (solution placed below my gums)
- ❏ Dietary counseling (education about my eating habits)
- ❏ Release of radiographs (x-rays) to the dentist of my choice, upon that dentist's request and/or my request
- ❏ Release of my dental hygiene records (periodontal and dental charting, record of services, etc.) to the dentist of my choice, upon the dentist's request or my request
- ❏ Intraoral photography (my identity will not be revealed)
- ❏ Other_____

I acknowledge that no guarantees have been made to me concerning the results of my dental hygiene care. Regardless of treatment, a risk of failure, relapse, or worsening of conditions may result. Adjunctive treatment or retreatment may be indicated. I recognize that long-term success depends on my cooperation, self-care practices, and routine maintenance. As treatment progresses, if alternative treatment is indicated, I expect the dental hygienist to discuss the additional treatment procedures.

I am aware that there are potential risks and consequences involved in any diagnostic, non-surgical, anesthetic, or analgesic procedure. Several potential risks include:

- ❏ Allergic reactions
- ❏ Excessive bleeding
- ❏ Gum recession exposing the root
- ❏ Infection
- ❏ Temporomandibular joint (TMJ) discomfort

- ❏ Pain
- ❏ Sensitivity
- ❏ Spaces between the teeth
- ❏ Temporary/permanent numbness
- ❏ Other_____

I have had all my questions answered. Knowing and understanding the treatment and risks, I consent to treatment.

- ❏ Option 1: As recommended.
- ❏ Option 2: As recommended, except _____

Client Signature:_____Clinician Signature:_____

Date of Consent:_____Date:_____

Sample Dialogs: A Practical Approach to Risk Management during Dental Hygiene Care

The following sample dialogs are provided to demonstrate the principles of communication presented on the CD ROMS.

SAMPLE DIALOG 1: NEED FOR LOCAL ANESTHESIA FOR DENTAL HYGIENE CARE

Clinician: The area I will be treating for you today is in the lower right quadrant which consists of these eight teeth (pointing to teeth). I realize from your medical history, and as I remember from previous discussions, you usually do not experience sensitivity. Is this still the case?

Patient: Usually. But sometimes it feels like you are scraping way down deep under my gums.

Clinician: That's a good observation; I probably was using my instruments in a "periodontal pocket"—an area that has lost bone support in the past. Today is another one of those days. Numbing the area is indicated to assure your comfort and allow me to feel that I can more thoroughly treat those periodontal pocket areas. What are your thoughts on local anesthesia?

Patient: That would be okay, but I'm surprised I need that this time. Are my teeth worse than before?

Clinician: No, not at all. The areas where you were uncomfortable on your previous appointments were these same areas that have more moderate pocket depths. The deeper the pocket, the more challenging it is for me to be able to thoroughly treat it while keeping you comfortable.

Patient: How many pockets do I have?

Clinician: There are six areas on the eight teeth that I will be debriding and root planing today. They are around your molars. Remember earlier today we looked at your x-rays and reviewed your oral hygiene in those areas. Knowing you will be comfortable throughout the procedure will make it easier for me to thoroughly treat the pockets and furcations we discussed.

Patient: I like the comfort idea.

Clinician: Since you've had injections before and we have discussed the risks associated with the administration of local anesthetic, I want to give you a chance to ask any questions you may have before I begin.

SAMPLE DIALOG 2: ANXIOUS PATIENT

Clinician: Thank you for sharing your childhood dental experiences with me. That injection would not have been pleasant for me either.

Patient: The needle hurt and it felt like my lip was swelling up really fast and there was a burning pain in my lip.

Clinician: It sounds like the injection was extremely uncomfortable for you. There are some techniques I can use to make the injection more comfortable. Are you the type of person who would be interested in hearing about these techniques or would you prefer not to?

Patient: It would be okay, just not the gory details.

Clinician: All right. I will apply topical anesthetic with a Q-tip to "numb" the area first and then I will proceed with the injection very slowly.

Patient: Will it hurt?

Clinician: No, it shouldn't. If you can take a couple of deep breaths to relax yourself, and I inject the anesthetic slowly, you will only feel a pinch for a second until the anesthetic enters your tissue and begins to numb the area.

Patient: It only takes a second?

Clinician: Let me clarify that statement. It only takes a second for the initial numbing of the tissue, but it will take a little longer for me to inject all of the solution. I assure you that it will make the injection much more comfortable if I proceed more slowly.

Patient: I'm still not excited about this, but I'll close my eyes and hold on tight until it is over.

Clinician: It's okay to close your eyes, but it would be more comfortable for you if you could try to relax by taking a couple of deep breaths rather than being tense. I also want you to know that if you need me to stop at any time just raise your left hand and I'll stop. (*Note:* the clinician may not really want to stop in the middle of the injection, but knowing that there is a choice in the situation offers the patient the feeling of maintaining some "control.")

Patient: That's good to know.

Clinician: Are you ready for me to start?

Patient: Okay.

SAMPLE DIALOG 3: INFORMED CONSENT WITH NEW PATIENT/NEW PROCEDURE

Clinician: I've reviewed your medical history very thoroughly and there doesn't seem to be any complication with our treatment today. You didn't have anything listed under chief concern today; is that correct?

Patient: Yes.

Clinician: (Clinician looks at the x-rays; notes areas of bone loss in the mandibular right quadrant; no incipient caries present.) Tell me about your previous experience at the dental office.

Patient: I've just had my teeth cleaned. I've never had a filling or a shot.

Clinician: From looking at your x-rays, it looks like you have taken care of your teeth throughout the years.

Patient: Yes, but I guess my gums are bad. They bleed when I brush them over here (pointing at the mandibular right quadrant).

Clinician: Well, they are not really bad. I can see from the x-rays some areas I will need to remove some calculus deposits and treat the roots of your teeth (pointing at that area on x-rays). Debridement/root planing procedures are a bit more extensive than a routine cleaning because we are providing nonsurgical therapy for the areas where your gums are infected and you have lost some bone support. Our goal is to arrest the disease process by treating those areas. And in order to do that and have it be more comfortable for you it is indicated that the area be numb.

Patient: Really?

Clinician: Yes. How do you feel about that?

Patient: I'm not sure.

Clinician: I'll go through the procedure and make sure you understand what I am going to do and that you agree to the treatment.

Patient: This is all different. I haven't had that either when I went to the dentist before.

Clinician: Well, since you have never had an injection it's important to me that you know the advantages, risks associated with administering local anesthetic, and those risks associated without the use of local anesthetic. After I go over these and you have a chance to ask questions, you will be better informed to give consent to the treatment.

Patient: All right.

Clinician: It is important to me that you understand any associated risks and that you have a voice in your treatment. The anesthesia will numb your teeth in that area (mandibular right quadrant), your tongue, and your lower lip for approximately 2 to 3 hours (*alter time depending on drug used, amount, etc.*).

Patient: That long?

Clinician: The numbness is minimal compared to the seemingly endless length of chair time for you if you are uncomfortable during the treatment.

Patient: I guess you are right, but nobody really likes the idea of a "shot."

Clinician: Let me remind you that risks associated with local anesthesia are minimal and extremely rare. They could include a slight temporary stiffness in the jaw or prolonged numbness in the area, some bruising in the area (hematoma), an allergic or toxic response, or some tissue sloughing at the site.

Patient: Wow, is it really risky?

Clinician: Remember the risks are minimal and extremely rare.

Patient: Okay.

Clinician: Also, you will need to be careful not to bite your lip or cheek while it is numb.

Patient: I know that. My son once traumatized his lip after he had a filling.

Clinician: Yes, that happens occasionally and can be uncomfortable. At the end of your appointment I will make sure to remind you to be careful when you bite until the anesthetic wears off. If we do not use anesthesia and you are uncomfortable during debridement/root planing, I cannot confidently treat the areas needing treatment. Then the chance of deposits remaining could be greater. If deposits remain in an area, the inflammation and bone loss we discussed might continue. (Pause.) Do you have any questions about anything I have discussed or have not discussed?

Patient: No, I can see the advantages.

Clinician: Is this treatment acceptable to you?

Patient: Yes.

Clinician: If at any time you feel any discomfort, please let me know by raising your left hand. I will also ask after treatment how you felt about today's appointment for future reference.

SAMPLE DIALOG 4: PATIENT WHO DECLINES/REJECTS INJECTION

Patient: I just came in to have my teeth cleaned and I don't need or want an injection.

Clinician: What you are saying is that you don't see the need for local anesthesia because most of your dental hygiene appointments in the past have been completed without injections?

Patient: Yes. I have had them for fillings but not when I had my teeth cleaned.

Clinician: After reviewing your chart and the x-rays it seems as though you have some areas where you have lost support to your teeth as a result of periodontal disease. Let me show you your x-rays and the tissue changes that have occurred in these areas. A "cleaning" or "prophylaxis" is indicated for prevention of your periodontal disease; it is no longer adequate once you have lost support. That's why I'm recommending nonsurgical periodontal therapy.

Patient: I know you explained that before but I'm not really clear on it.

Clinician: Let me try to make myself clearer. We not only remove plaque, toxins, and calculus deposits but also treat root surfaces and tissue in pocket areas to allow them to heal and arrest progressing disease and infection. The procedure is called periodontal debridement/root planing and it is often performed with local anesthesia to assure comfort in these areas. Without anesthesia it could be uncomfortable for you.

Patient: That's a given.... I've never had a comfortable time in the dental office!

Clinician: That's unfortunate. Your previous dental appointments seem to have been very unpleasant.

Patient: You have that right! I don't know why it's so miserable for me.

Clinician: Dental and dental hygiene care does not have to be uncomfortable. I'd like to discuss with you some techniques that would lessen the discomfort during your dental hygiene appointment.

Patient: If these techniques have to do with a needle I don't want to hear about it.

Clinician: You sound dead set against an injection whether it decreases your discomfort or not. Why is that?

Patient: I just don't like the needle. It hurts worse than the cleaning or filling itself.

Clinician: If we don't use anesthesia, and you are uncomfortable during the treatment, I in turn will be less confident treating you, and the chance of deposits remaining may be greater. If the deposits remain in the area, the inflammation and bone loss might continue.

Patient: I understand but I still do not want an injection.

Clinician: Okay. I'm not here to force you into anything. I will begin debridement/root planing in the area and you can stop me at any time and we can revisit the option of numbing the area if you decide you want to.

Patient: I won't need it.

Clinician: So you don't have to go through this at your next dental hygiene appointment I will make a note in your chart stating you declined to have local anesthetic during this dental hygiene appointment and what we discussed today.

Patient: Okay, thanks.

Summary of Postexposure Protocol

• Cleanse wound	Wash the wound and skin that contacted the blood or body fluids with soap and water; flush mucous membranes with water.
• Explain to patient what has occurred and OSHA (Occupational Safety and Health Administration) guidelines for postexposure testing	Discuss the proper protocol to follow, according to the policies of the individual workplace. Good communication skills are imperative in this situation.
• Obtain patient consent for testing	Arrange for source patient testing, if the source is known and consents to testing.
• Set up immediate testing appointment for exposed worker and for patient— as soon as possible following exposure	Health care providers who evaluate the exposed worker should be: • Selected *before* Dental Health Care Workers (DHCW) are placed at risk of exposure • Experienced in providing antiretroviral therapy • Familiar with the unique nature of dental injuries so they can provide appropriate guidance on the need for antiretroviral prophylaxis

(continued)

• Fill out occupational incident form (see Sample Exposure Report/Questionnaire	Employers should follow all federal and state requirements for recording and reporting occupational injuries and exposures. The incident report should include: • Date and time of exposure • Details of the procedure being performed, including where and how the exposure occurred and, if the exposure was associated with a sharp device, the type of device and how and when in the course of handling the device the exposure occurred • Details of the exposure, including the type and amount of fluid or material and the severity of the exposure (e.g., for a percutaneous exposure, depth of injury and whether the fluid was injected; for a skin or mucous-membrane exposure, the estimated volume of material as well as the duration of contact and condition of the skin) • Details about the exposure source (i.e., whether the source material contained HIV or other blood-borne pathogens) and, if the source is HIV positive, the stage of disease, history of antiretroviral therapy, and viral load, if known; details about counseling, postexposure management, and follow-up • Details about the exposed person (e.g., hepatitis B virus vaccine and vaccine-response status) • Details about counseling, postexposure management, and follow-up
• Written report/opinion of health-care provider	Within 15 days of evaluation, the qualified health-care provider sends a written opinion to the employer. The report contains only: • Documentation that the employee was informed of evaluation results and the need for further follow-up • Whether hepatitis B (HBV) vaccine was indicated and if it was received All other findings are confidential and are not included in the report.
Employer informs employee (DHCW)	The employer keeps a copy of the health-care provider's written report on file in confidential medical record, and provides a copy of written opinion to exposed employee.

Refer to http://www.ada.org/prof/resources/topics/osha/intro.asp for additional information.

Sample Exposure Report/Questionnaire

The following forms are available through the CDC and can be modified to reflect your specific clinical needs.

EXPOSED EMPLOYEE INFORMATION

Name_____   Social Security No._____   Job Title_____

Employer Name_____   Address_____

Time the injury occurred_____   Time reported_____   Date_____

Has the employee received HBV?   ❏ Yes   ❏ No

If "Yes": Dates of vaccination 1._____   2._____   3._____

Post-vaccination HBV antibody status, if known:_____   Positive_____   Titer_____

Negative_____   Unknown_____

Date of last tetanus vaccination:_____

Review of exposure incident follow-up procedures: ❏ Yes This form completed by

_____

EXPOSURE INCIDENT INFORMATION

Is the injury sharps related?   ❏ Yes   ❏ No

If "Yes,": Type of sharp_____   Brand_____

Work area where exposure occurred:_____

Procedure in progress:_____

How incident occurred:_____

Location of exposure (e.g., "right index finger"):

Did sharps involved have engineered injury protection?   ❏ Yes   ❏ No

If "Yes": Was the protective mechanism activated? ❏ Yes   ❏ No

The injury occurred (circle one) BEFORE / DURING / AFTER activation of protective mechanism.

If "No": In the employee's opinion, could a mechanism have prevented the injury: ❏ Yes   ❏ No

If so, how?_____

In the employee's opinion, could any engineering, administrative, or work practice control have prevented the injury?   ❏ Yes   ❏ No

Explain:

SOURCE PATIENT INFORMATION

Name_____   Chart No._____

Telephone No:_____

Consent to release of information to evaluating health-care professional   ❏ Yes   ❏ No

Patient Signature:_____

Review of source patient medical history   ❏ Yes   ❏ No

Verbally questioned regarding:

History of hepatitis B, hepatitis C, or HIV infection   ❏ Yes   ❏ No

If HIV-positive, antiretroviral medication history:

High-risk history associated with these diseases   ❏ Yes   ❏ No

Patient consents to be tested for HIV, hepatitis C, and hepatitis B virus   ❏ Yes   ❏ No

EVALUATING HEALTH-CARE PROFESSIONAL INFORMATION

Referred to (name of evaluating health-care worker):_____

Questionnaire completed by:_____

Bill for fees to:

_____

Retain one copy in employee's confidential medical record; send one copy to evaluating health-care professional with the exposed dental worker.

Centers for Disease Control Screening Form

INSTRUCTIONS FOR USING THE SAMPLE SCREENING FORM

Adapting the Form

The form can be modified to reflect your specific clinical needs by adding criteria that reflect your practice or deleting criteria that are not appropriate for your practice. For example, if your patient population consists primarily of children, you may choose to add criteria that reflect the use of the device in small mouths.

Completing the Form

In the screening phase, include a representative of each type of dental personnel that will be using or handling the device. Be sure that each person completing the form has a sample of the safer device as well as the traditional device in front them.

Interpreting the Results

Once the form has been completed by all personnel, discuss the results to determine whether to proceed to the next phase—evaluating the safer device in the clinical setting. In making this decision, some criteria may be more important than others. For example, clinical and safety feature considerations may be more important than the general product (e.g., availability of the device) or practical considerations (e.g., instructions and packaging). If the responses to many criteria are "Does Not Meet Expectations" or "No," then you should consider other safer devices; otherwise, evaluate the device in the clinical setting.

Sample Screening Form—Dental Safety Syringes and Needles

This form collects the opinions and observations of dental healthcare personnel who screen a safer dental device to determine its acceptability for use in a clinical setting. This form can be adapted for use with multiple types of devices. **Do not use a safer device on a patient during this initial screening phase.**

Date:_____

Product: Name, brand, company:_____

Your position or title:_____

Your occupation or specialty:_____

CLINICAL CONSIDERATIONS	DOES NOT MEET EXPECTATIONS	MEETS EXPECTATIONS	EXCEEDS EXPECTATIONS
1. The device permits the exchange of cartridges during treatment on the same patient.	1	2	3
2. The weight and size of device is acceptable.	1	2	3
3. I have a clear view of the cartridge contents when aspirating.	1	2	3
4. The size and configuration of the syringe or needle permits a clear view of the injection site and needle tip.	1	2	3
5. No excessive force is required to activate or control the plunger.	1	2	3
6. The size and configuration of the syringe or needle permits use in all mouth sizes and access to all areas of the mouth.	1	2	3
7. The device permits multiple injections on the same patient.	_____ No	_____ Yes	
8. The device is capable of aspiration before injection.	_____ No	_____ Yes	
9. The needle is compatible with a reusable syringe. [For safety needles without syringes only.]	_____ No	_____ Yes	
Does the product meet the needs of your clinical practice based on the above criteria?	_____ No	_____ Yes	
10. The worker's hands can remain behind the sharp during activation of the safety feature.	1	2	3

SAFETY FEATURE CONSIDERATIONS	DOES NOT MEET EXPECTATIONS	MEETS EXPECTATIONS	EXCEEDS EXPECTATIONS
11. The safety feature can be activated with one hand.	1	2	3
12. The safety feature is integrated into the syringe or needle.	1	2	3
13. The safety feature provides a temporary means of protecting the needle between injections.	1	2	3
14. A visible or audible cue provides evidence of safety feature activation.	1	2	3
15. The safety feature is easy to recognize and use.	_____ No	_____ Yes	

(continued)

SAFETY FEATURE CONSIDERATIONS	DOES NOT MEET EXPECTATIONS	MEETS EXPECTATIONS	EXCEEDS EXPECTATIONS
16. Once activated, the safety feature permanently isolates the needle tip and cannot be purposefully or accidentally deactivated under normal use conditions.	_____ No	_____ Yes	
17. The safety feature activates by itself.	_____ No	_____ Yes	

GENERAL PRODUCT/MANUFACTURE CONSIDERATIONS

18. The manufacturer can provide the device in needed quantities.	1	2	3
19. A full range of needle sizes and lengths is available.	1	2	3
20. The company provides free samples for in-use evaluation.	1	2	3
21. The company has a history of responsiveness to problems.	1	2	3

PRACTICAL CONSIDERATIONS

22. The device is packaged conveniently.	1	2	3
23. The device is easy to remove aseptically from the package.	1	2	3
24. Instructions are included in the packaging.	1	2	3
25. Instructions are easy to follow and complete.	1	2	3
26. Instructions are provided in more than one form (paper, videotape, Web site, or computer disk).	1	2	3
27. Use of the safety device will not increase the volume of sharps waste.	1	2	3
28. The shape and size of available sharps containers will accommodate disposal of this device.	1	2	3
29. This is a single use, disposable device.	_____ No	_____ Yes	
30. The device should be considered for further clinical evaluation.	_____ No	_____ Yes	

Additional comments for any responses of "Does Not Meet Expectations " or "No":

_____

_____

_____

Sample Device Evaluation Form—Dental Safety Syringes and Needles

INSTRUCTIONS FOR USING THE SAMPLE DEVICE EVALUATION FORM

Adapting the Forms

Like the screening form, the device evaluation form can be modified to reflect your clinical needs by adding criteria that reflect your practice or by deleting criteria that are less relevant to your practice.

Obtaining Feedback

Select staff who represent the scope of personnel who will use or handle the device. Choose a reasonable testing period—2 to 4 weeks should be sufficient. Staff should receive training in the correct use of the device, which can often be provided by product representatives. Encourage staff to provide informal feedback during the evaluation period. Monitor the pilot test to ensure proper use of the safer device and remove the device immediately if it is found to be unsafe. Forms should be completed and returned to the safety coordinator as soon as possible after the evaluation period.

Interpreting the Results

After the evaluation phase, speak with personnel who have completed the forms to determine the criteria that should receive the most consideration. For example, personnel may express that criteria regarding the "feel" of the device (e.g., weight and size of the device, how the device fits in their hand) are important in maintaining proper injection technique. If the responses to many of the criteria are "Strongly Disagree" or "Disagree," check with personnel who have completed the form to obtain additional information. Balance this feedback with safety and practical considerations before determining whether to continue using the device in your practice.

SAMPLE DEVICE EVALUATION FORM
DENTAL SAFETY SYRINGES AND NEEDLES

This form collects opinions and observations from dental healthcare personnel who have pilot tested a safer dental device. This form can be adapted for use with multiple types of safer devices. Do not use this form to collect injury data because it cannot ensure confidentiality.

Date:_____

Product: Name, brand, company:_____

Number of times used: _____

Your position or title:_____

Your occupation or specialty:_____

1. Did you receive training in how to use this product?

   ❏ Yes [Go to Next Question]   ❏ No [Go to Question 4]

2. Who provided this instruction? (Check All that Apply.)

   ❏ Product representative   ❏ Staff member   ❏ Other

3. Was the training you received adequate?

   ❏ Yes   ❏ No

4. Compared to others of your sex, how would you describe your hand size?

   ❏ Small   ❏ Medium   ❏ Large

5. What is your sex?   ❏ Female   ❏ Male

Please answer all questions that apply to your duties and responsibilities. If a question does not apply to your duties and responsibilities, **please leave it blank.**

DURING THE PILOT TEST OF THIS DEVICE . . .	STRONGLY DISAGREE	DISAGREE	NEITHER AGREE NOR DISAGREE	AGREE	STRONGLY AGREE
6. The weight of the device was similar to that of a conventional dental syringe.	1	2	3	4	5
7. The device felt stable during assembly, use and disassembly.	1	2	3	4	5
8. The device fit my hand comfortably.	1	2	3	4	5
9. The anesthetic cartridges were easy to change.	1	2	3	4	5
10. Aspiration of blood into the anesthetic cartridge was clearly visible.	1	2	3	4	5
11. I had a clear view of the injection site and needle tip.	1	2	3	4	5
12. The device did not appear to increase patient discomfort.	1	2	3	4	5
13. The device performed reliably.	1	2	3	4	5
14. I was able to give injections in all mouth sizes and all areas of the mouth.	1	2	3	4	5
15. I used the device for all of the same purposes for which I use the conventional device.	1	2	3	4	5
16. Activating the safety feature was easy.	1	2	3	4	5
17. The safety feature was easy to recognize and use.	1	2	3	4	5

(continued)

DURING THE PILOT TEST OF THIS DEVICE . . .	STRONGLY DISAGREE	DISAGREE	NEITHER AGREE NOR DISAGREE	AGREE	STRONGLY AGREE
18. The safety feature did not activate inadvertently, causing me to use additional syringes or needles.	1	2	3	4	5
19. The safety feature functioned as intended.	1	2	3	4	5
20. The instructions were easy to follow and complete.	1	2	3	4	5
21. I could have used this product correctly without special training.	1	2	3	4	5
22. The "feel" of the device did not cause me to change my technique.	1	2	3	4	5
23. This device meets my clinical needs.	1	2	3	4	5
24. This device is safe for clinical use.	1	2	3	4	5

Additional comments for any responses of "Strongly Disagree " of "Disagree."

_____

_____

_____

_____

SECTION IV LEARNING ACTIVITIES

1. Call 3-5 offices and inquire what their policies are on the following: Sharps disposal (location & number of containers; method of container disposal), needlestick policy, compliance with OSHA policy on evaluating needle safety devices, informed consent policy (written vs. verbal).

2. Observe a peer/colleague and evaluate his/her communication skills (both verbal and nonverbal) before, during, and after the administration of local anesthesia. (NOTE: refer to the *Communications Assessment* form for evaluation criteria).

   Before: Obtaining informed consent

   During: while administering injection

   After: written documentation. Were all required elements/items included in the written record?

3. Evaluate Written Documentation: Randomly select, review and evaluate 5 recent local anesthesia chart entries from patient files. What is missing? What corrections should be made to assure documentation is complete and accurate?

4. EBDM: Conduct an evidence-based review to determine the most current OSAP and CDC needlestick policies. What are they? What are the OSHA regulations that have developed as a result of these guidelines?

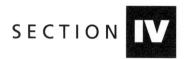

Risk Management/Quizz

Communication, Informed Consent, Documentation, Occupational Exposures Self-Test

SECTION **4-1 to 4-4**

1. The single most important factor ("the *key*") to avoiding medicolegal complications is:
   a. Knowledge of current information and techniques
   b. Good technical skills
   c. Effective communication skills
   d. Obtaining written informed consent
   e. Thorough knowledge of Occupational Safety and Health Administration (OSHA) regulations
   f. Securing an attorney with expertise in dental litigation

2. The following characteristics are critical to successful clinician/patient relationship:
   1. Respect
   2. Adherence
   3. Empathy
   4. Cohesiveness
   5. Warmth

   Answer:
   a. 1 only
   b. 1 and 4
   c. 1, 2, and 3
   d. 1, 3, and 5
   e. All of the above

3. Which of the following types of behaviors are considered to be nonverbal?
   1. Body orientation
   2. Voice tone
   3. Active listening
   4. Paraphrasing
   5. Eye contact

   Answer:
   a. 1 and 2
   b. 1 and 5
   c. 3 and 5
   d. 1, 3, and 5
   e. 1, 4, and 5
   f. All of the above

4. For which of the following reasons does paraphrasing facilitate communication between the patient and clinician?
   1. The listener has an avenue to repeat what was seen or heard
   2. Each party has the opportunity to correct any misconceptions
   3. It prevents miscommunication
   4. It increases the accuracy of the message
   5. It clarifies the verbal message, but not the nonverbal message

   Answer:
   a. 1 and 2
   b. 3 and 5
   c. 1, 2, and 4
   d. 3, 4, and 5
   e. 1, 2, 3, and 5

5. Which of the following is an example of demonstrating empathy?
   a. Acknowledgment of the patient's feelings
   b. Acknowledgement of associated risks
   c. Effective eye contact
   d. Proper body orientation
   e. Use of soft voice

6. Paraphrasing allows the clinician (or patient) to summarize what has been seen or heard, allowing both parties to verify both verbal and nonverbal behaviors.
   a. The first part of the statement is true, the second part is false
   b. The first part of the statement is false, the second part is true
   c. Both parts of the statement are true
   d. Both parts of the statement are false

7–9. Matching: Fill in the blank with the principle for improving listening comprehension that corresponds with the example.
   Principles:
   a. Pay attention to nonverbal behavior
   b. Periodically review and summarize what is being said
   c. Anticipate where the conversation is going
   d. Objectively weigh the information being presented by the patient

7. _____ Mentally consider what the patient is trying to tell you

8. _____ Paraphrase verbal and nonverbal behaviors to patient for reaction

9. _____ Patient is observed as fidgeting in chair, perspiring

10. A message of five sentences or longer without allowing a response is considered cooperative communication between an oral health professional and patient.
    a. True
    b. False

11. Because dental hygienists, in most cases, practice under the supervision of a licensed dentist, they are not exposed to risk management issues.
    a. True
    b. False

12. A dental hygienist practicing in a state where local anesthesia is a delegable procedure is more accountable for his or her actions than is a dental hygienist practicing in a state where the administration of local anesthesia is not a legal procedure for hygienists.
    a. True
    b. False

13. Applying proper communication techniques can be just as important to successful treatment as other "technical" skills.
    a. True
    b. False

14. Most dental education programs include intensive study in the area of human behavior.
    a. True
    b. False

15. Generally speaking, patients prefer to know what is going to happen during each appointment.
    a. True
    b. False

16. Any time treatment is recommended, it is essential not only that the patient be given the information about the treatment, risks, and alternatives, but also that the patient understands the information.
    a. True
    b. False

17. Given all pertinent information, the patient makes the decision whether or not to proceed with the procedure.
    a. True
    b. False

18. Potential treatment risks are discussed after treatment has been completed.
    a. True
    b. False

19. Verbal acceptance of treatment by the client is acceptable; however, a signed document is preferable for obtaining informed consent.
    a. The first part of the statement is true, the second part is false
    b. The first part of the statement is false, the second part is true
    c. Both parts of the statement are true
    d. Both parts of the statement are false

20. When obtaining informed consent, what information must be provided to the patient? (check all that apply—no partial credit will be given).
    a. Explanation of the treatment recommended
    b. Optional treatment plan(s)
    c. Potential risks
    d. Consequences of not pursuing treatment
    e. Associated fees
    f. Opportunity for the patient to ask questions
    g. Educational background of providers

21. It is recommended that clients be involved when the clinician is documenting their dental hygiene care.
    a. True
    b. False

22. Should litigation occur or a suit proceed to court, the jury would be asked to determine whether the patient was informed of risks associated with no treatment.
    a. True
    b. False

23. The longer the written entry in the patient's record, the less chance litigation might occur.
    a. True
    b. False

24. When documenting a patient's behavior, limit the use of verbs. Quoting the patient's exact words and corresponding behavior is recommended.
    a. The first statement is true, the second is false
    b. The first statement is false, the second is true
    c. Both statements are true
    d. Both statements are false

25. According to OSHA, PEP is the acronym for:
    a. Professional Employees Protection
    b. Personal Exposure Protection
    c. Post Exposure Prophylaxis
    d. Protected Employee Plan
    e. Personal Equipment Protection

26. According to the U.S. Public Health Service (PHS) the preferred method for dealing with occupational exposures is prevention.
    a. True
    b. False

27. Following the administration of an injection, the clinician improperly recaps the needle and accidentally sticks herself with the contaminated needle. She immediately cleanses the wound. According to current occupational exposure guidelines, what is the next most appropriate course of action to follow?
    a. Document the exposure event on appropriate OSHA form(s)
    b. Call an attorney to seek counseling regarding the occupational exposure
    c. Discuss the incident with the patient, obtaining permission and making arrangements for blood testing
    d. Dismiss the patient and reschedule the appointment for 3 days subsequent to the blood test(s)

28. After a syringe is used on a patient, which of the following is the best methods for the clinician to make the needle safe?
    a. Pass the syringe to an assistant to put away
    b. Place syringe on a tray and dispose after patient treatment
    c. Scoop cap that has been lying on tray onto needle and leave until treatment is completed
    d. Bend the needle at the plastic syringe adaptor with hemostat and place in sharps container

29. What procedure should a clinician follow if accidentally stuck by a needle after it has been used on a patient?
    a. Report the incident to the local health board
    b. Have the patient sign a statement regarding AIDS status
    c. Follow protocol mandated by national/state OSHA regulations
    d. Tell supervising dentist and have him or her fill out appropriate paperwork

30. The placement of well-designed sharps container is not a concern, as long as they are clearly marked and recognizable to workers.
    a. True
    b. False

Nitrous Oxide/Oxygen Analgesia

Nitrous Oxide and Oxygen Flowmeters

Following are examples of nitrous oxide (N_2O) and oxygen flowmeters and the likely settings used when administering appropriate sedation levels during the incremental induction technique.

1. Beginning sedation with oxygen at 5 to 7 Lpm: adjust individual's need by observing reservoir bag. In this example, the liters per minute is set at 5.

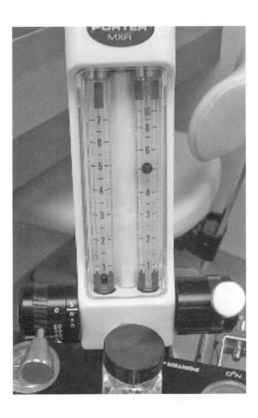

2. The flowmeter has been adjusted to approximately 10% to 15% N$_2$O—some individuals may begin to feel effects at this level.

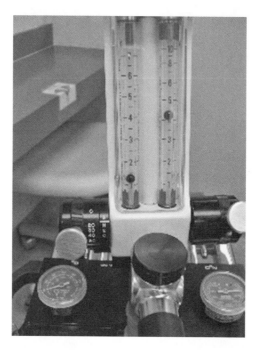

Remember as you change each setting, the total flow (combined N$_2$O and oxygen) should be kept at the same liters per minute of oxygen your patient started on at beginning of sedation—5 Lpm in this example.

3. The flowmeter has been adjusted to approximately 20% to 25% N$_2$O: Suggest symptoms and explain safety of mouth breathing if uncomfortable sensations occur.

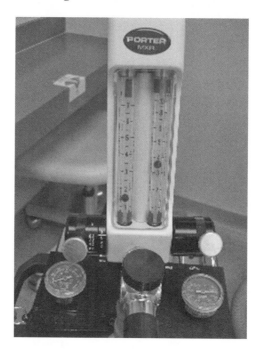

4. In this photo the flowmeter has been adjusted to approximately 35% N₂O. Most individuals reach appropriate sedation levels between 25% and 45%.

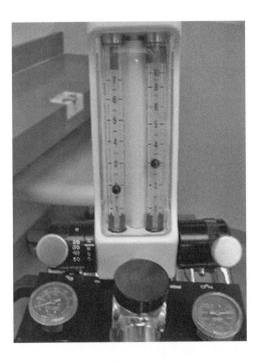

5. The flowmeter has been adjusted to approximately 50% N₂O in this photo. Very few individuals require more than 50%. Check tubing, mouth breathing, etc. if sedation level is not achieved at this setting.

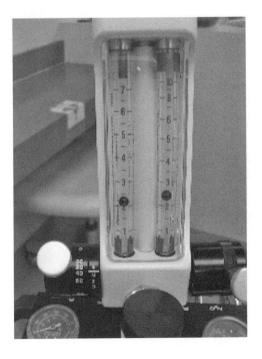

Summary of Recommendations and Contraindications

NITROUS OXIDE

Nitrous oxide is a conscious sedation drug that allows for exact titration (incremental administration) for individual patient needs, has a rapid onset of sedation (1 to 5 min), a rapid emergence from sedation (3 to 5 min), and has a high analgesic effect. Nitrous oxide sedation helps to overcome patient fear and pain.

Indication for use: mild pain, control fear or anxiety, gag reflex, long treatment time, local anesthetic not wanted or tolerated. (Note: Should never try to replace local anesthetic with nitrous oxide.)

The information in the following charts for Section V was compiled primarily from Berthold (2002), Clark (2003), Haas (1999), Jackson (2002), and Malamed (2003).

NO CONTRAINDICATIONS	POSSIBLE CONTRAINDICATIONS	ABSOLUTE CONTRAINDICATIONS
Cardiovascular system (CVS): Myocardial infarction, atherosclerosis, heart murmur, congenital sond; rheumatic fever, angina, surgery-valve bypass, transplant, hypertension, bleeding diathesis **Central nervous system (CNS):** Stroke, seizure disorders, fainting spells, Parkinson disease **Respiratory system:** Patients with asthma—positive relaxing **Hematopoietics:** Anemias, methemoglobinemia, sickle-cell anemia, leukemia, hemophilia, polycythemia vera **Hepatic system:** Hepatitis, jaundice **Endocrine system:** Diabetes, thyroid/adrenal dysfunction **Kidney disease:** Okay; no negative effects of N_2O **Neuromuscular system:** Multiple sclerosis, muscular dystrophy, cerebral palsy, myasthenia gravis **Cancer:** Positive analgesic, sense of well-being **Allergies:** No known reported allergies within 150 years (other than latex related) **Drug interactions:** no direct interaction with N_2O, but enhances effect of CNS depressants	• Sinus infection, congestion—postpone N_2O treatment • Bronchitis, chronic or episodic—consult medical doctor • Tuberculosis (TB), upper respiratory infections—postpone N_2O treatment • Ear infections—medical doctor consult or postpone N_2O treatment • Mental illness, retardation, Alzheimer disease, autism—discretion and medical doctor consult • Bowel obstructions—postpone N_2O treatment • Debilitating cardiac disease—not recommended • Those taking CNS depressants (morphine, alcohol, etc.)—intensifies N_2O effect • HIV/AIDS—not recommended if in later stage • Recovered alcoholic or history of drug abuse—not recommended • Pregnancy—consult medical doctor • Claustrophobia	• Chronic obstructive pulmonary disease (COPD)/emphysema "O_2-driven," hypoxic-driven respiration—not recommended, hypoxic due to lack of respiratory drive • Cystic fibrosis • Recent ophthalmic surgery • Pneumothorax—postpone treatment until resolved • Latex allergy (if equipment is made with rubber materials) and equipment is made with rubber materials

Summary of Sedation Levels and Patient Symptoms

STAGES OF SEDATION

Stage I Analgesia/Sedation
Stage III Planes of Surgical Anesthesia

Stage II Excitement/Delirium
Stage IV Medullary Paralysis/Death

STAGE I (PLANES 1, 2, 3)—PLANES 1 AND 2 *MOST* DESIRABLE FOR DENTAL TREATMENT	STAGE II *NOT* RECOMMENDED FOR DENTAL TREATMENT
• Patient feels happy, relaxed, comfortable, aware of surroundings; responds rationally, reduced sense of anxiety, fear, pain • Patient may get a glazed or twinkling look, big smile • Tingling fingers, toes, cheeks, head, and lips • Heaviness in legs, followed by floating • Voice changes, warmth and flushed feelings • Patients should be questioned specifically about "what" they feel not "how" they feel because varying degrees of any or all symptoms may be experienced • Titrate N_2O until relaxed/comfortable • Up to 50% N_2O minimum 30% O_2	• All effects intensify or disappear; some continue to be pleasant • *Changes occur rapidly* • Increased N_2O levels become uncomfortable, closely monitor and be prepared to decrease N_2O immediately • Patient becomes lightheaded, dizzy, speech impaired, nausea, restless, hot, possibly combative or violent, agitated • Eyes fixed, panic • Excitement phase begins
STAGE III SURGERY ANESTHESIA *NOT* RECOMMENDED	**STAGE IV**
• Hallucinations, nausea, vomiting, excitation, nonresponsive • Unconsciousness • Eyes dilated • Life threatening	• Medullary paralysis • Death

PATIENT SYMPTOMS

IDEAL PATIENT SYMPTOMS	INAPPROPRIATE SYMPTOMS
• Relaxed • Happy, comfortable. and aware of surroundings • Responds rationally and coherently • Reduced sense of anxiety and fear • Dreamy look • Tingling in extremities • Slight ringing in ears • Heaviness or lightness in arms/legs • Warm and drowsy/slightly flushed • Vital signs normal	• Closes mouth frequently • Patient unaware of surrounding • Hallucinations • Dilation of pupils • Excitation/hard stare • Agitated or combative

(continued)

REPORTED SIDE EFFECTS	TOXICITY
Nausea with high or prolonged exposures, potential negative psychological response with mental illness, possible diffusion hypoxia and headaches In high concentration: hallucinations, hypnosis, general anesthesia, sexual phenomena, crying, laughing (excessive), extended euphoria	Insignificant or nonexistent if used on a healthy patient carefully titrated to receive only the amount of N_2O needed to reach a relaxed comfortable state of sedation and used for reasonable lengths of time Negative experiences associated with inappropriate amounts of N_2O

Summary of Technique Instructions

NITROUS OXIDE SEDATION INDUCTION TECHNIQUES

Incremental Induction Technique

- Medical History Evaluation
- With patient in supine position:
  - Establish tidal volume—start at 6 L 100% oxygen
  - Watch reservoir bag to evaluate need to increase or decrease tidal volume
  - Allow patient to ask any questions verbally now
- At 1 min of 10% nitrous oxide—suggest patient may start feeling effects; remind patient to breathe deeply
- At 1 min of 20% nitrous oxide—explain possible symptoms: warmth, relaxation, paresthesia
  - Explain safety of mouth breathing—If patient feels dizzy/nauseous they can breathe through their mouth
- At 1 min of 25% nitrous oxide
  - Continue to suggest symptoms
  - Average patient reaches appropriate sedation between 25% and 45% N_2O
- Continue at 5% increments until any of the symptoms are present. If 50% nitrous oxide is reached with no symptoms, check mouth breathing, shallow breathing, loose mask, kinking of tubing
- Ask patient to take three deep breaths and adjust flow rates accordingly
- Continue at 5% increments. Monitor carefully—very few patients need more than 50% nitrous oxide. Maximum limit 70%
- Following sedation give 100% oxygen for 3 to 5 min to flush nitrous oxide from respiratory system. Allow patient to recover sitting upright to avoid hypotension.
- Determine complete recovery before releasing patient from office

Rapid Induction Technique

- Must know patient's usual percentage of N_2O
- Establish tidal volume from records or a new level with 100% O_2
- Administer 70% N_2O at 10 L/min and have the patient take **three deep breaths**
- Collapse the bag by hand to express all the contents
- Administer usual N_2O percentage and reduce flow to normal tidal volume for patient
- Patient will notice effect within a few breaths

This is a very dramatic and quick technique and should be used with caution; not appropriate for all patients.

Calculation of Nitrous Oxide/Oxygen Chart

PERCENTAGES OF N_2O/O_2

LITERS PER MIN. N_2O	LITERS PER MINUTE OF O_2									
	1	2	3	4	5	6	7	8	9	10
1	50	33	25	20	17	14	13	11	10	9
2	67	50	40	33	29	25	22	20	18	17
3	75*	60	50	43	38	33	30	27	25	23
4	80*	67	57	50	44	40	36	33	31	29
5	83*	71	63	56	50	45	42	38	36	33
6	86*	75*	67	60	55	50	46	43	40	38
7	88*	78*	70	64	58	54	50	47	44	41
8	89*	80*	73	67	62	57	53	50	47	44
9	90*	82*	75*	69	64	60	56	53	50	47
10	91*	83*	77*	71	67	63	59	56	53	50

*Percentage exceeds maximum amount of N_2O needed for effective pain/anxiety management in an ambulatory setting and exceeds amounts able to be delivered by analgesia machines.

Example calculation if chart is not available

What is the percentage of N_2O if patient is receiving 4 L of O_2 and 3 L of N_2O?

4 + 3 = 7 L total flow

3 (liters of N_2O) ÷ 7 (total Lpm) = 43% N_2O

Summary of Standards for Maintenance and Control of Nitrous Oxide Equipment

STEP BY STEP APPROACH FOR CONTROLLING N_2O/O_2

STEP	PROCEDURE	CONTROL
1	Visually inspect all N_2O equipment (reservoir bag, hoses, mask, connectors) for worn parts, cracks, holes, or tears.	Replace defective equipment and/or parts.
2	Turn on the N_2O tank and check all high- to low-pressure connections for leaks. Use a non-oil-based soap worn solution to check for bubbles at high-pressure connectors, or use a portable infrared gas analyzer.	Determine leak source and fix. If tank valve leaks, replace tank; if O-rings, gaskets, valves, hoses, or fittings, replace. Contact the manufacturer for parts for parts replacement. For threaded pipe fittings, use Teflon tape. Do not use this tape on compression fittings.
3	Select scavenging system and mask. Mask should come in various sizes to patients. Scavenging systems should operate at airflow rate of 45 Lpm	Provide a range of mask sizes for patients. Check to see that noise levels at the mask are acceptable when the scavenging system exhaust rate is operated at 45 Lpm.
4	Connect mask to hose and turn on vacuum pump before turning on N_2O. Scavenging system vacuum pump must have capacity to scavenge 45 Lpm per dental operation.	Determine proper vacuum pump size for maintaining 45 Lpm flow rates, especially when interconnected with other dental scavenging systems. If undersized, replace pump.
5	Place mask on patient and assure a good, comfortable fit. Make sure reservoir bag is not over- or underinflated while the patient is breathing.	Secure mask with "slip" ring for "good activity" from patient breathing.
6	Check general ventilation for good room air mixing. Exhaust vents should not be close to air supply vents (use smoke tubes to observe air movement in room).	If smoke from smoke tubes indicates room air mixing is poor, then increase the airflow or redesign. If exhaust vents are close to air supply vents, relocate (check with ventilation engineers to make adjustments).
7	Conduct personal sampling of dentist and dental assistant for N_2O exposure. Use diffusive sampler or infrared gas analyzer (see sampling methods).	If personal exposures exceed 150 ppm during administration, improve mask fit and make sure it is secure over the patient's nose. Minimize patient talking while N_2O is administered.

(continued)

STEP	PROCEDURE	CONTROL
8	Repeat procedure in step 7.	If personal exposures are less than 150 ppm but greater than 25 ppm, implement auxiliary exhaust ventilation near the patient's mouth. Capture distance should no greater than 10 in. from the patient's nose and mouth area and exhaust no less than 250 cfm (cubic foot per minute) at the hood opening. Avoid getting between the auxiliary exhaust hood and patient's mouth and nose area.

This information is taken from DHHS (NIOSH) Publication No. 96–107.

N_2O/O_2 SEDATION RECORD (SAMPLE FORM)

Date:_____   Patient:_____   Age:_____

ASA Classification: I   II   III   IV

Med Consult needed?:   Yes/No   If yes, describe results_____

_____

_____

_____

Treatment Procedure: _____

Procedural Data:

PREOPERATIVE   POSTOPERATIVE
_____

BP _____   _____

Pulse/Quality _____   _____

Respiration _____   _____

N_2O start time _____ N_2O finish time _____

Total Flow (liters/minute) _____

Titrated % of N_2O _____ Postoperative O_2 (in minutes) _____

Comments:

_____

_____

_____

_____

_____

_____

Clinician Signature: _____

SECTION V LEARNING ACTIVITIES

1. Use the sample Nitrous Oxide/Oxygen Evaluation Form (included in *Supplementary Clinical Manual*) to self-assess your administration technique.

2. Call 3-5 offices and inquire what their policies are on:
   a. equipment maintenance, for example: checking gas levels in the tanks, checking leaks in the hoses/reservoir bag, scavenging system, method of monitoring ambient gas levels, frequency of maintenance
   b. administration, for example: patients that are contraindicated to receive nitrous in their office, titration technique, who may administer nitrous in their office, for how long are patients oxygenated following administration, informed consent and written documentation policies.

3. Using the checklist provided from NIOSH (included in *Supplementary Clinical Manual*), check the equipment in your office for controlling nitrous oxide exposure levels.

4. Review statutes in your state for rules and regulations regarding nitrous oxide administration and monitoring. Be aware of which members of the dental team can administer and/or monitor nitrous oxide/oxygen and specific guidelines for legal compliance in your state.

5. Determine percentage of nitrous oxide and oxygen levels for each of the following scenarios:
   a. Your patient is receiving 4 liters of O_2 and 3 liters of N_2O.
      _____% of Nitrous Oxide
      _____% of Oxygen
   b. Your patient is receiving 3 liters of O_2 and 2 liters of N_2O
      _____% of Nitrous Oxide
      _____% of Oxygen
   c. Your patient is receiving 5 liters of O_2 and 1 liter of N_2O
      _____% of Nitrous Oxide
      _____% of Oxygen

6. What are some of the items a patient may list on their medical history that may be a possible contraindication for the administration of nitrous oxide?

7. EBDM: Identify and discuss the controversy regarding NIOSH guidelines regarding the limit of 50 ppm nitrous oxide gas in the dental operatory.

Nitrous Oxide/Oxygen Sedation/Quizzes

1. Which of the following is a characteristic of nitrous oxide?
   a. Nitrous oxide is stored in the body
   b. Nitrous oxide is a sweet-smelling, colorless gas
   c. Nitrous oxide is easily titrated
   d. Patients may be allergic to nitrous oxide
   e. b and c

2. Nitrous oxide is used in which areas of medicine?
   a. Dentistry
   b. Obstetrics
   c. Podiatry
   d. a and b
   e. All of the above

3. The optimum level of nitrous oxide is what percentage?
   a. 5%
   b. 10%
   c. 25%
   d. 50%
   e. Depends on the individual patient's signs and symptoms

4. What would the gauge read on a half full cylinder of oxygen?
   a. 325 psi
   b. 500 psi
   c. 750 psi
   d. 1000 psi
   e. 2000 psi

5. The nitrous oxide tank, in the US, is what color?
   a. White
   b. Blue
   c. Green
   d. Gray
   e. Red

6. The reservoir bag monitors which of the following?
   a. patient's respirations
   b. Flow of nitrous oxide
   c. Flow of oxygen
   d. The need to adjust the liters per minute flow of gases
   e. a and d

7. For which of the following patients may nitrous oxide be contraindicated?
   a. Recovered alcoholic
   b. Person taking central nervous system sedatives
   c. Emphysema
   d. b and c
   e. All of the above

8. Which of the following reactions would indicate that a patient is *not* being maintained at the appropriate level of relative analgesia?
   a. The patient giggles
   b. The patient has a "floating" feeling
   c. The patient has slight ringing in the ears
   d. The patient's pupils are dilated
   e. The patient feels a slight tingling in the fingers and toes

9. Delivery of nitrous oxide to a patient with which one the following conditions maybe contraindicated?
   a. Anemia
   b. Diabetes
   c. Ear infection
   d. Hepatitis
   e. High blood pressure

10. How are the patient's vital signs affected by administration of nitrous oxide at the appropriate levels of sedation?
   a. Pulse is accelerated; respiration and blood pressure remain unchanged
   b. Pulse, respiration, and blood pressure are all lowered significantly
   c. Pulse, respiration, and blood pressure remain within normal range
   d. Pulse is reduced; blood pressure and respiration remain unchanged
   e. Blood pressure, respiration, and pulse are all accelerated

11. Which of the following conditions may contraindicate the administration of nitrous oxide?
   a. Severe chronic obstructive pulmonary disease
   b. Hypertension or cardiovascular disease
   c. Psychiatric disorders
   d. a and c
   e. All of the above

12. A scavenging system should vacuum exhaled gases at how many liters per minute to be effective?
   a. 6 to 7 Lpm
   b. 12 to 15 Lpm
   c. 25 Lpm
   d. 45 Lpm
   e. 75 Lpm

13. At 50% nitrous oxide the patient states he is not feeling much effect. What should you do?
   a. Check nose piece to see if there is a seal around the nose
   b. Keep increasing the level by 10% per minute to see if effect increases
   c. Check hoses to see if there are any kinks
   d. a and c
   e. All of the above

14. Why does nitrous oxide have a very rapid onset?
    a. It fills the lungs up to capacity very rapidly
    b. The bloodstream absorbs the nitrous oxide completely
    c. Very little of nitrous oxide is absorbed into the bloodstream
    d. It diffuses across the pulmonary tissues very slowly
    e. b and d

15. How many liters of air does a normal adult inhale per minute?
    a. 2 to 3
    b. 3 to 5
    c. 5 to 8
    d. 10 to 12
    e. 12 to 15

16. Effects of adequate sedation may include which of the following?
    a. Relief of anxiety
    b. Tingling of the extremities
    c. Warm, flushed feeling
    d. a and b
    e. All of the above

17. Which of the following may indicate the patient has diffusion hypoxia after nitrous oxide is discontinued?
    a. Very high blood pressure
    b. Headache
    c. Lethargy
    d. b and c
    e. All of the above

18. Which of the following items may cause fire or explosion when working with nitrous oxide?
    a. Oil around the valves of the oxygen tank
    b. Grease around the nitrous oxide tank
    c. Lack of copper tubing used to distribute gases from the tanks
    d. b and c
    e. All of the above

19. What are the current recommendations by the National Institute for Occupational Safety and Health (NIOSH) for acceptable parts per million (ppm) of nitrous oxide in the dental office?
    a. 35 ppm
    b. 40 ppm
    c. 45 ppm
    d. 50 ppm
    e. A level has not been established by NIOSH

20. At what level should you begin the administration of nitrous oxide?
    a. 5%
    b. 10%
    c. 15%
    d. 20%
    e. 25%

21. Most patients will achieve the desired clinical level of sedation at what percent of nitrous oxide?
    a. 10% to 20%
    b. 15% to 20%
    c. 25% to 45%
    d. 45% to 50%
    e. Usually over 50%

22. If you were using a central supply nitrous oxide sedation system, which of the following components would you have that would not be used on a portable unit?
    a. Multiple flowmeter heads
    b. Larger cylinders
    c. Copper pipes
    d. a and b
    e. All of the above

23. Where is most of the nitrous oxide metabolized/eliminated in the body?
    a. In the lungs
    b. In the liver
    c. In the kidneys
    d. In the gastrointestinal tract
    e. All of the above

24. Which of the following may contraindicate the use of nitrous oxide sedation?
    a. Sinus infection
    b. In patients with cancer
    c. Bowel obstructions
    d. a and c
    e. All of the above

25. If you are delivering 4 L of oxygen and 3 L of nitrous oxide to your patient, what is the percent of nitrous oxide being delivered?
    a. 25%
    b. 33%
    c. 43%
    d. 50%
    e. 70%

Key to Quizzes/Self Tests

Pain/Nerve Conduction SECTION 1-1

1	b	10	a	19	b
2	b	11	a	20	c
3	d	12	e	21	b
4	c	13	d	22	c
5	a	14	b	23	d
6	c	15	b	24	b
7	b	16	c	25	a
8	b	17	c		
9	a	18	b		

Types and Action of Local Anesthetic Agents SECTION 1-2

1	d	5	a	9	c
2	d	6	e	10	a e b c d
3	e	7	e	11	a
4	e	8	a		

Pharmacology of Local Anesthetics SECTION 1-3

1	b	5	b	9	c
2	b	6	e	10	e
3	c	7	b		
4	b	8	a		

Pharmacology of Vasoconstrictors

1	c	5	b	9	c
2	d	6	d	10	b
3	c	7	a		
4	c	8	e		

Selection of Local Anesthetic Agents

1	e	8	a	15	a
2	c	9	e	16	d
3	a	10	b	17	b
4	d	11	b	18	d
5	d a c e b	12	a	19	c
6	d	13	c	20	b
7	c	14	a		

Trigeminal Nerve

1		5	b	14	b
a.	Superior Orbital fissure	6	Lingual nerve	15	b
b.	Foramen Rotundum	7	Inferior alveolar nerve	16	a
c.	Foramen Ovale	8	Buccal Nerve	17	a
d.	Ophthalmic	9	Sphenomandibular ligament	18	e
e.	Maxillary			19	b
f.	Mandibular	10	f b g a e d c	20	b
2	c	11	b	21	b
3	d	12	e		
4	b	13	a		

Armamentarium

1	a	8	b	15	a	
2	f	9	c	16	30 gauge	
3	c	10	e	17	27 gauge	
4	b	11	d	18	*	
5	e	12	aspirating	19	red	
6	e	13	c	20	after 3-4 uses on 1 pt.	
7	h	14	b and g			

*18. it's impossible to tell from the cap (unless it is a short cap and then it's obviously a short needle). The color coded cap indicates gauge only—not length.

Technique

1	c	10	a	19	medial pterygoid muscle
2	a	11	d	20	d
3	b	12	c	21	b
4	c	13	d	22	b
5	a	14	b	23	d
6	d	15	i	24	b
7	a	16	d	25	b
8	b	17	c		
9	b	18	a		

Selection of Injections

1	a	5	a	9	d
2	b	6	a	10	e
3	d	7	c		
4	c	8	b		

Alternatives

1	e		5	d		9	e
2	c		6	e		10	d
3	b		7	b			
4	c		8	e			

Physical Evaluation

1	d		5	c		9	b
2	e		6	b		10	e
3	c		7	e		11	d
4	c		8	c		12	a

Complications

1	b		6	a		11	b
2	b		7	c		12	d
3	h		8	a		13	d
4	b		9	c		14	e
5	b		10	c		15	c

Risk Management

1	c		5	a		9	a
2	d		6	c		10	b
3	b		7	c		11	b
4	c		8	b		12	b

13	a	19	c	25	c
14	b	20	a b c d e f	26	a
15	a	21	a	27	c
16	a	22	a	28	c
17	a	23	b	29	c
18	b	24	b	30	b

Nitrous Oxide

SECTION **5-1 to 5-5**

1	c	10	c	19	d
2	e	11	d	20	b
3	e	12	d	21	c
4	d	13	d	22	e
5	b	14	c	23	a
6	e	15	c	24	d
7	e	16	e	25	c
8	d	17	d		
9	c	18	e		

REFERENCES

SECTION I. LOCAL ANESTHETIC AGENTS

American Dental Association Guide to Dental Therapeutics. 3rd ed. Chicago, IL: ADA Publishing Division; 2003.

ADA/PDR Guide to Dental Therapeutics. 4th ed. Thomas Healthcare; 2006.

American Dental Association Council on Dental Education. *Guidelines for Teaching the Comprehensive Control of Pain and Anxiety in Dentistry.* Adopted by ADA house of Delegates; Oct. 2003.

Bare L, Dundes M. Strategies for combating dental anxiety. *J Dent Educ.* 2004;68(11).

Bay N, Cannon TM. Management of the fearful patient. *J Dent Hyg.* 1990;64(5):188–191.

Bennett CR. *Monheim's Local Anesthesia and Pain Control in Dental Practice.* 7th ed. St. Louis, MO: C.V. Mosby; 1984.

Bouffard C. *Controlling Pain and Anxiety.* Access; April 1999.

Clark M, Brunick A. *Handbook of Nitrous Oxide and Oxygen Sedation.* 2nd ed. St. Louis, MI: Mosby; 2003.

Clinical Research Associates Newsletter (CRA). June 2005;29(6).

Hass D. An update on local anesthetics in dentistry. *J Canad Dent Assoc.* 2002;68(9).

Evers H, Haegerstam G. *Introduction of Local Anaesthesia.* 2nd ed. Philadelphia, PA: BC Decker Inc.; 1990.

Fehrenbach MJ. *Pain Control in Dental Hygiene,* RDH, February 2005.

Finder RL, Moore PA. Adverse drug reactions to local anesthesia. *Dent Clin North Am.* Oct. 2002;46(4).

Fiset L, Leroux B, et al. Pain control in recovering alcoholics: effects of local anesthesia. *J Stud Alcohol.* May 1997;58.

Gadbury-Amyot CC, Overman PR, Carter-Hanson C, et al. An Investigation of Dental Hygiene Treatment Fear. *J Dent Hyg.* 1996;70(3).

Gadbury-Amyot CC, Williams KB. Dental hygiene fear: gender and age differences. *J Contemp Dent Pract.* 2000;1(2).

Hass DA. An update on local anesthetics in dentistry. *J Canad Dent Assoc.* 2002;68(9).

Hawkins JM, More PA. Local anesthesia: advances in agents and techniques. *Dent Clin North Am.* 2002;46.

Hodges KOH, ed. *Concepts in Nonsurgical Periodontal Therapy.* Albany, NY: Delmar; 1998.

Jastak JT, Yagiela JA, et al. *Local Anesthesia of the Oral Cavity.* Philadelphia, PA: W.B. Saunders; 1995.

Lipp, Markus DW. *Local Anesthesia in Dentistry.* Carol Stream, IL: Quintessence Publishing; 1993.

Little JW, Falace DA, et al. *Dental Management of the Medically Compromised Patient.* 6th ed. St. Louis, MI: Mosby; 2002.

Maggirias J, Locker D. Psychological factors and perceptions of pain associated with dental treatment. *Commun Dent Oral Epidemiol.* 2002;30.

Malamed SF. *Sedation: A Guide to Patient Management.* 3rd ed. St. Louis, MI: Mosby; 1995.

Malamed SF. *Handbook of Local Anesthesia.* 5th ed. St. Louis, MO: C.V. Mosby; 2004.

Malamed SF. Up close with amide anesthetic agents. *Dimensions of Dental Hygiene.* June 2005.

Malamed SF. All about vasoconstrictors. *Dimensions of Dental Hygiene.* September 2005.

McCann D. Dental phobia: conquering fear with trust. *J Am Dent Assoc.* 1989;119.

Meechan JG. *Practical Dental Local Anaesthesia.* London: Quintessance Publishing; 2002.

Meechan JG, Rood JP. Adverse effects of dental local anesthesia. *Dental Update.* October 1997;24.

Meit SS, Yasek V, et al. Techniques for reducing anesthetic injection pain. *J Am Dent Assoc.* September 2004;135.

Milgrom P, Weinstein P, Kleinknecht R, et al. *Treating Fearful Dental Patients.* Reston, VA: Reston Publishing Company; 1995.

Milgrom P, Coldwell SE, et al. Four dimensions of fear of dental injections. *J Am Dent Assoc.* June 1997;128.

Miller-Keane Encyclopedia and Dictionary of Medicine, Nursing and Allied Health. 5th ed, Philadelphia, PA: WB Saunders; 1992.

Moore PA. Adverse drug in dental practice: interactions associated with local anesthetics, sedatives and anxiolytics. *J Am Dent Assoc.* April 1999; 130.

Naftalin LW, Yagelia JA. Vasoconstrictors: indications and precautions. *Dent Clin North Am.* October 2002;46(4).

Pallasch, T. Vasoconstrictors and the heart. *CDA J.* September 1998;26(9).

Robinson PD, Ford TR, et al. *Local Anaesthesia in Dentistry.* Edinburgh, Wright/Elsevier; 2000.

Rowe MM. Dental fear and HIV contagion. *J Practical Hygiene.* September–October 1997.

Seeley R, Stephens T, Tate P. *Anatomy & Physiology.* 6th ed. St. Louis, MI: Mosby; 2004.

Smith T, Heaton M. Fear of dental care: are we making any progress? *J Am Dent Assoc.* August 2003;134.

Sohn W, Ismail A. Regular dental visits and dental anxiety in an adult dentate population. *J Am Dent Assoc.* January 2005;136.

Sullivan MJL, Neish NR. Psychological predictors of pain during dental hygiene treatment. *Probe: J Canad Dent Hygienists Assoc.* 1997;31:4.

Wahl M. Local anesthetics and vasoconstrictors: myths and facts. *Oral Pathology.* 1997;9(6).

Wahl MJ, Schmitt MM, et al. Injection pain of bupivacaine with epinephrine vs. prilocaine plain. *J Am Dent Assoc.* December 2002;133.

Wynn RL, Bergman SA, Meiller TF. Paresthesia associated with local anesthetics: a perspective on articaine. *Gen Dent.* November–December 2003;51(6).

Yagiela JA. Adverse drug interactions in dental practice: interaction associated with vasoconstrictors. *J Am Dent Assoc.* May 1999;130.

Zubieta J, et al. Can't stand the pain? Your genes may be to blame. *Science.* February 2003.

Young ER, MacKenzie TA. The pharmacology of local anesthetic agents: a review of the literature. *J Canad Dent Assoc.* 1992;58(1);34–42.

SECTION II. INJECTIONS

Agur AM, Dalley AF. *Grant's Atlas of Anatomy.* 11th ed. Baltimore, MD: Lippincott, Williams & Wilkins; 2005.

American Dental Association Council on Dental Education. *Guidelines for Teaching the Comprehensive Control of Pain and Anxiety in Dentistry.* Adopted by ADA house of Delegates, October 2003.

American Dental Hygiene Association. *Administration of Local Anesthesia by Dental Hygienists State Chart.* April 2005.

AGD Impact. *Local Injection Gone Awry.* February 2002.

Bassett K, McIntosh K. *Local Anesthesia,* Dimensions of Dental Hygiene, March 2005.

Bay N, Cannon TM. Management of the fearful patient. *J Dent Hyg.* 1990;64(5):188–191.

Bennett CR. *Monheim's Local Anesthesia and Pain Control in Dental Practice.* 7th ed. St. Louis, MO: C.V. Mosby; 1984.

Blanton PL, Jeske AH. Misconceptions . . . involving local anesthesia. *Texas Dent J.* April 2002;119(4).

Blanton PL, Jeske AH. The key to profound anesthesia neuroanatomy. *J Am Dent Assoc.* 2003;134.

Blanton PL, Jeske AH. Dental local anesthetics alternative delivery methods. *J Am Dent Assoc.* February 2003;134.

Blanton PL, Jeske AH. Avoiding complications in local anesthesia induction. *J Am Dent Assoc.* July 2003;134.

Burns Y. Reader A, et al. Anesthetic efficacy of the palatal-anterior superior alveolar injection. *J Am Dent Assoc*. September 2005;35.

Chamberlain TM, Davis RD, et al. Systemic effects of an intraosseous injection of 2% lidocaine with 1:100,000 epinephrine. *Gen Dent*. May–June 2000;48(3).

Cook-Waite Anesthetics from Kodak Dental Products, *Prescribing Information*. New York, 1993:1–9.

Clinical Research Associates Newsletter, Clinicians Guide to Dental Products and Techniques. Articaine HCL 4% with epinephrine 1:100,000 – update '05. June 2005;29(6).

Costa CG, Tortamano IP, et al. Onset and duration periods of articaine and lidocaine on maxillary infiltration. *Quintessence Int*. March 2005;36(3).

Crout RJ, Koraido G, Moore PA. A clinical trial of long-acting local anesthetics for periodontal surgery. *Anesthesia Progress*. 1990;37(7).

CRA Foundation. Oraqix – Significant anesthesia without injection. *Dental Hygiene Newsletter*. May–June 2005;5(3).

Dower JS. A review of paresthesia in association with administration of anesthesia. *Dentistry Today*. 2003;22(2).

Evers H, Haegerstam G. *Introduction of Local Anaesthesia*. 2nd ed. Philadelphia, PA: BC Decker Inc.; 1990.

Fehrenbach MJ. *Pain Control in Dental Hygiene*. RDH, February 2005.

Fehrenbach MJ. *Gow-Gates Mandibular Nerve Block: An Alternative in Local Anesthetic Use*. Access; November 2002.

Friedman MJ. New advances in local anesthesia. *Compendium*. 2000;21(5):432–440.

Friedman MJ, Hochman MN. A 21st century computerized injection system for local pain control. *Compendium*. 1997;18(10):995–1003.

Fukayma H, Yoshikawa F, et al. Efficacy of anterior and middle superior alveolar (AMSA) anesthesia using a new injection system: The Wand. *Quintessance Int*. 2003;34(7).

Gallatin J, Reader A. A comparison of two intraosseous anesthetic techniques in mandibular posterior teeth. *J Am Dent Assoc*. November 2003;134.

Haas DA, Lennon D. A 21 year retrospective study. *J Canad Dent Assoc*. 1995;61(4).

Hawkins JM. *Articaine:Truths Myths and Potentials*. Academy of Dental Therapeutics and Stomatology. Vol 9, 2003.

Hawkins JM, Moore PA. *Local Anesthesia: Advances in Agents and Techniques*. Dental Clinics of North America. Vol 46, 2002.

Hiatt JL, Gartner LP. *Textbook of Head and Neck Anatomy*. 3rd ed. Philadelphia, PA: Lippincott, Williams and Wilkins; 2002.

Houchman MN, Friedman MJ. In vitro study of needle deflection: a linear insertion technique versus a bidirectional rotation insertion technique. *Quintessence Int*. 2000;31(1).

Houchman MN, Friedman MJ. An in vitro study of needle force penetration comparing a standard linear insertion to the new bidirectional rotation insertion technique. *Quintessence Int*. 2001;32(10).

Houpt MI, Heins P, et al. An evaluation of intraoral lidocaine patches in reducing needle-insertion pain. *Compendium*. 1997;18(4):309–316.

Jastak JT, Yagiela JA, Donaldson D. *Local Anesthesia of the Oral Cavity*. Philadelphia, PA: C.V. Mosby; 1995.

Jeffcoat MK, Geurs NC, et al. Intrapocket anesthesia for scaling and root planing: results of a double-blind multicenter trial using lidocaine and prilocaine gel. *J Periodontol*. July 2001;72(7).

Kennedy S, Reader A, The significance of needle deflection in success of the inferior alveolar nerve block in patients with irreversible pulpitis. *J Endodontics*. October 2003;29(10).

Kleber CH. Intraosseous anesthesia implications, instrumentation and techniques. *J Am Dent Assoc*. April 2003;134.

Leonard MS. The efficiency of an intraosseous injection. *J Am Dent Assoc.* 1995;126.

Loomer PM, Perry DA. Computer-controlled delivery versus syringe delivery of local anesthetic injections for therapeutic scaling and root planning. *J Am Dent Assoc.* March 2004;135.

Lipp MDW. *Local Anesthesia in Dentistry.* Carol Stream, IL: Quintessence Publishing;1993.

Madan GA, Madan SG. Failure of inferior nerve block: exploring the alternatives. *J Am Dent Assoc.* July 2002;133.

Magnusson I, Jeffcoat MK, et al. Quantification and analysis of pain in nonsurgical scaling and/or root planning. *J Am Dent Assoc.* December 2004;135.

Malamed SF. *Handbook of Local Anesthesia.* 5th ed. St. Louis, MO: C.V. Mosby;2004.

Malamed SF, Gagnon S, et al. Efficiency of articaine: new amide anesthetic. *J Am Dent Assoc.* 2000;131.

Malamed SF, Gagnon S, et al. Articaine hydrochloride: a study of the safety of a new amide local anesthetic. *J Am Dent Assoc.* February 2001;132.

Martin EJ. *No Pain, All Gain? Electronic Dental Anesthesia Tries To Take Charge.* AGD Impact; April 1996.

Meecham JG. *Practical Dental Local Anaesthesia.* London: Quintessance Publishing; 2002.

Meechan JG, Gowans AJ, et al. The use of patient-controlled transcutaneous electronic nerve stimulation (TENS) to decrease the discomfort of regional anaesthesia in dentistry : a randomized conrolled clinical trial. *J Dentistry.* July–August 1998;26(5–6).

Meit SS, Yasek V, et al. Techniques for reducing anesthetic injection pain. *J Am Dent Assoc.* September 2004;135.

Milgrom P, Weinstein P, Kleinknecht R, et al. *Treating Fearful Dental Patients. A Patient Management Handbook.* Reston, Virginia: Reston Publishing Company; 1985.

Moore KL, Dalley AF. *Clinically Oriented Anatomy.* 4th ed. Baltimore, MD: Lippincott, Williams & Wilkins; 1999.

Moore PA. Adverse drug interactions in dental practice: interactions associated with local anesthetics, sedatives and anxiolytics. *J Am Dent Assoc.* April 1999;130.

Nusstein JL, Reader A, et al. Injection pain and postinjection pain of the anterior middle superior alveolar injection administered with the Wand or conventional syringe. *Oral Surg Oral Med Oral Pathol Oral Radiol Endod.* July 2004;98(1).

Organization of Safety and Asepsis Procedures (OSAP). Achieving OSHA Compliance, Rules and regulations for the dental office. July 2002;1(2).

Quarnstrom F, Libed EN. Electronic anesthesia versus topical anesthesia for the control of injection pain. *Quintessence Int.* October 1994;25(10).

Quinn JH. Inferior Alveolar Nerve Block Using The Internal oblique Ridge, *J Am Dent Assoc.* August 1998;129.

Robinson PD, Ford TR, et al. *Local Anaesthesia in Dentistry.* Edinburgh, Wright/Elsevier;2000.

Rosenberg ES, A Computer-Controlled Anesthetic Delivery System in a Periodontal Practice: Patient Satisfaction and Acceptance, *J Esthet Restor Dent.* 2002;14(1).

Seeley R, Stephens T, Tate P. *Anatomy & Physiology.* 6th ed. New York: McGraw-Hill Science/Engineering/Math; 2003.

Trebus DL, Singh G, et al. Anatomical basis for inferior alveolar nerve block, *Gen Dent.* November–December 1998.

Wong JK, Adjuncts to local anesthesia: separating fact from fiction, *J Canand Dent Assoc.* 2001;67.

Yagiela JA. Recent developments in local anesthesia and oral sedation. *Compendium.* September 2004;25(9).

SECTION III. POTENTIAL COMPLICATIONS

American Dental Association Guide to Dental Therapeutics. 3rd ed. Chicago, IL: ADA Publishing Division; 2003.

ADA/PDR Guide to Dental Therapeutics. 4th ed. Thomas Healthcare; 2006.

America Society of Anesthesiologists. New classification of physical status. *Anesthesiology.* 1963; 24:111.

Aubertin MA. The hypertensive patient in dental practice: updated recommendations for classification, prevention, monitoring and dental management, *J Gen Dent.* November–December 2004.

Balicer RD, Kitai E. Methemoglobinemia caused by topical teething preparation: a Case Report. *Scientific World Journal.* July 15, 2004.

Baluga, JC. Allergy to local anesthetics in dentistry: myth or reality? *Rev Alerg Mex.* September–October 2003; 50(5).

Bennett CR. *Monheim's local anesthesia and pain control in dental practice.* 7th ed. S. Louis, MO: C.V. Mosby; 1984.

Brion CR. *Adverse Reactions to Local Anesthetics.* RDH October 2000.

Blanton BL, Jeske AH. Avoiding complications in local anesthesia induction. *J Am Dent Assoc.* July 2003;134.

Budenz AW. *Local Anesthetics and Medically Complex Patients, J Calif Dent Assoc.* August 2000; 28(8).

Campbell JR, Maestrello CL, et al. Allergic response to metabisulfite in lidocaine anesthetic solution. *Anesthesia Progress.* 2001;48.

Carmona IT, Diz Dios P, Scully C. An update on the controversies in bacterial endocarditis of oral origin. *Oral Surg Oral Med Oral Pathol Oral Radiol Endod.* June 2002;93(6).

Chen AH. Toxicity and allergy to local anesthesia. *Calif Dent Assoc.* September 1998;26(9).

Finder RL, Moore PA. Adverse drug reactions to local anesthesia. *Dent Clin North Am.* October 2002;46(4).

Faura-Sole M. Sanchez-Garces MA, et al. Broken anesthetic injection needles: Report of 5 cases. *Quintessence Int.* 1999;30.

Hass DA. An update on local anesthetics in dentistry. *J Canadi Dent Assoc.* 2002;68(9).

Hass DA. Localized complications from local anesthesia. *Calif Dent Assoc.* September 1998;26(9).

Jainkittivong A, Aneksuk V, Langlais RP. Medical health and medication use in elderly dental patients. *J Contemporary Dental Practice.* February 2004;5(1).

Herman WW, Konzelman JL. New national guidelines on hypertension: A summary for dentistry. *J Am Dent Assoc* May 2004;135.

Lessard E, Glick M, et al. The patient with a heart murmer evaluation, assessment and dental considerations. *J Am Dent Assoc.* March 2005;136.

Little JW, Falace DA, et al. Dental Management of the Medically Compromised Patient. 6th ed. St. Louis, MI: Mosby; 2002.

Little J. The American Heart Association's guidelines for the prevention of bacterial endocarditis: a critical review. *Gen Dent.* September–October 1998;46(5).

Malamed SF. *Handbook of Local Anesthesia.* 5th ed. St. Louis, MO: C.V. Mosby;2004.

Malamed SF. *Medical Emergencies in the Dental Office.* 5th ed. St. Louis, MI: Mosby;2000.

Malamed SF. All About Vasoconstrictors. Dimensions of Dental Hygiene; September 2005.

Meechan JG. Rood JP. Adverse effects of dental local anesthesia, dental update. Department of Oral and Maxillofacial Surgery, University of Newcastle upon Tyne October 1997;24.

Meechan JG. *Practical Dental Local Anaesthesia.* London: Quintessance Publishing; 2002.

Milzman DP, Milzman JB. Treatment of patients with medical considerations and complications. *Dent Clin North Am.* July 1999;43(3).

Naftalin LW, Yagelia JA. Vasoconstrictors: indications and precautions, *Dent Clin North Am.* October 2002;46(4).

Pallasch TJ. Antibiotic prophylaxis: problems in paradise. *Dent Clin North Am.* October 2003;47(4).

Pallasch T. Vasoconstrictors and the heart. *CDA J.* September 1998;26(9).

Pickett F, Gurenlian J. *The Medical History: Clinical Implications and Emergency Prevention in Dental Settings.* Baltimore, MD: Lippincott Williams and Wilkins; 2005.

Pogrel MA, Schmidt BL, et al. Lingual nerve damage due to inferior alveolar nerve blocks, *J Am Dent Assoc.* February 2003;134.

Pinto A, Glick M. Management of patients with thyroid disease, oral health considerations. *J Am Dent Assoc.* July 2002;133.

Ring T. *Diabetes: An Epidemic on the Rise.* Access; July 2001.

Spolarich AE. *Drugs Used to Manage Cardiovascular Disease.* Access; March 2001.

Spolarich AE. *The Top 20 Most Commonly Prescribed Medications for 2004.* Access; December 2005.

U.S. Department of Health and Human Services, National Institutes of Health; National Heart, Lung and Blood Institute, National Blood Pressure Education Program. The seventh report of the Joint National Committee on Prevention, Detection, Evaluation and Treatment of High Blood Pressure, April 2004, Available at www.nhlbi.nih.gov/guidelines/hypertension/indes.htm

Wahl M. Local anesthetics and vasoconstrictors: myths and facts. *Oral Pathol.* 1997;9(6).

Wilburn-Goo D, Lloyd LM. When patients become cyanotic: acquired methemoglobinemia. *J Am Dent Assoc.* June 1999;130.

Yagiela JA. Adverse drug interactions in dental practice: interaction associated with Vasoconstrictors. *J Am Dent Assoc.* May 1999;130.

Zhang C, Banting DW, et al. Effect of B-adrenoreceptor blockade with nadolol on the duration of local Anesthesia. *J Am Dent Assoc.* December 1999;130.

SECTION IV. RISK MANAGEMENT

American Dental Association Council on Insurance. Informed consent: a risk management view. *J Am Dent Assoc.* 1987;115:632.

American Dental Association Department of State Government Affairs. Personal correspondence; 1998.

American Dental Association Website: http://www.ada.org/prof/resources/topics/osha/intro.asp

Bennett CR. *Monheim's Local Anesthesia and Pain Control in Dental Practice.* 7th ed. St. Louis, MO: C.V. Mosby; 1984:24.

Bolton R. *People Skills.* New York City, NY: Simon & Schuster; 1979:36.

Bressman JK. Risk management for the 90's. *J Am Dent Assoc.* 1993;124:64–67.

Centers for Disease Control and Prevention (CDC) Website: www.cdc.gov/OralHealth/infection-control/index.htm

Darby ML. *Comprehensive Review of Dental Hygiene Care.* 4th ed. St. Louis, MO: C.V. Mosby; 1998:767.

David J. *People Factor Training Manual & Guide.* St Petersburg, FL: INNERSEE; 1987:6.

De Jongh A, Stouthard MEA. Anxiety about dental hygienist treatment. *Community Dent Oral Epidemiol.* 1993;21:91–95.

D'Eramo E. The office anesthesia record. *J Am Dent Assoc.* 1979;98:407–409.

DeVore CH. Legal risk management for the dental hygienist. *J Prac Hyg.* 1997;6(4):59–61.

Freeman R. Reflections on professional and lay perspectives of the dentist-patient interaction. *Br Dent J.* 1999;186(11):546–550.

Gadbury-Amyot C. An investigation of dental hygiene treatment fear. *J Dent Hyg.* 1996;70(3):115–121.

Garza GM, Childers WC, Walters RP. *Interpersonal Communication.* Gaithersburg, MD:Aspen Publishers; 1982:163.

Graskemper JP. Informed Consent: A stepping stone in risk management. *Compendium.* 2005; 26(4):286–290.

Hodges KOH, ed. *Concepts in Nonsurgical Periodontal Therapy.* Albany, NY: Delmar Publishers; 1998:524.

Mears P. *Healthcare Teams: Building Continuous Quality Improvement.* Delray Beach, FL: St. Lucie Press; 1994:5.

Milgrom P, Weinstein P, Kleinknecht R, et al. *Treating Fearful Dental Patients.* Reston, VA: Reston Publishing Company, Inc.; 1995:15.

Molinari JA. Risks and prevention of occupational exposures: role of sharps containers. *J Prac Hyg.* November–December 1998.

National Institute for Occupational Safety and Health (NIOSH) Website: http://www.cdc.gov/niosh/2000-108.html

Office Safety and Asepsis Procedures (OSAP) Research Foundation. *Postexposure Prophylaxis: CDC Issues Recommendations for Healthcare Workers Exposed to HIV,* Focus #5, 1998.

Orr DL, Curtis WJ. Obtaining written informed consent for the Administration of Local Anesthetic in Dentistry. *J Am Dent Assoc.* November 2005;136.

OSAP: Dentistry's Resource for Infection Control and Safety. *From Policy to Practice: OSAP's Guide to the Guidelines.* Annapolis, MD: Office Safety and Asepsis Procedures (OSAP); 2004.

Office Safety and Asepsis Procedures (OSAP) Website: http://www.osap.org/

OSHA Website: http://www.osha.gov/SLTC/dentistry/index.html

Public Health Service. Guidelines for the management of health-care worker exposures to HIV and recommendations for postexposure prophylaxis. 1998;05:15.

Purton C. *Person-Centered Therapy: The Focusing-Oriented Approach.* New York City, NY: Palgrave MacMillan; 2004.

Sullivan MJL, Neish NR. Psychological predictors of pain during dental hygiene treatment. *Probe J.* 1997;31(4):123–126.

Van Servellen G. *Communication Skills for the Health Care Professional Concepts and Techniques.* Gaithersburg, MD: An Aspen Publication; 1997.

SECTION V. NITROUS OXIDE/OXYGEN SEDATION

Agur MR, Dalley AF, *Grants Atlas of Anatomy.* 11th ed. Philadelphia, PA: Lippincott, Williams & Wilkins; 2005.

American Dental Association Guidelines for the Use of Conscious Sedation, Deep Sedation and General Anesthesia for Dentists. Adopted by the American Dental Association House of Delegates, October 2003.

American Academy of Pediatric Dentistry Council on Clinical Affairs. Policy on minimizing occupational health hazards associated with nitrous oxide. *Pediatr Dent.* 2005–2006;27(7 reference manual): 49–50.

American Dental Association Guide to Dental Therapeutics. 3rd ed. Chicago, IL: ADA Publishing Division; 2003.

American Dental Association Website (ada.org). Position papers.

American Dental Hygiene Association Website (ADHA.org). Current data/chart on States which allow administration and/or monitoring of nitrous oxide sedation by auxiliaries.

America Society of Anesthesiologists. New classification of physical status. *Anesthesiology.* 1963;24:111.

Berthold M. Safety alert: nitrous oxide screen for recent ophthalmic surgery. *Am Dent Assoc News.* May 2002.

Clark M, Brunick A. *Handbook of Nitrous Oxide and Oxygen Sedation.* 2nd ed. St. Louis, MI: Mosby; 2003.

Clark M, Renehan B, Feffers B. Clinical use and potential biohazards of nitrous oxide/oxygen. *Gen Dent.* September–October 1997.

Certosimo F, Walton M, et al. Clinical evaluation of the efficiency of three nitrous oxide scavenging units during dental treatment. *Gen Dent.* September–October 2002;50(5)

Darby ML, Walsh MM. *Dental Hygiene Theory and Practice.* 2nd ed. St. Louis, MI: Saunders; 2003.

Department of Health and Human Services (NIOSH) Publication No. 96–107

Donaldson D. *Nitrous Oxide Sedation Video.* Canada: University of British Columbia; 1990.

Donaldson D, Garbi J. The efficiency of nitrous oxide scavenging devices in dental offices. *J Can dent Assoc.* July 1989;55:7.

Encyclopedia & Dictionary of Medicine, Nursing and Allied Health. 5th ed. Philadelphia, PA: W.B. Saunders; 1992.

Haas DA. Oral and inhalation conscious sedation anesthesia in dentistry. *Dent Clin North Am.* April 1999;43:2.

Holroyd I, Roberts GJ. Inhalation sedation with nitrous oxide: a review. *Dent Update.* April 2000;27(3).

Howard W, Nitrous oxide in the dental environment: assessing the risk, reducing the exposure. *J Am Dent Assoc.* March 1997;128.

Jacobs S, Haas D, et al. Injection pain comparison of three mandibular block techniques and modulation by nitrous oxide:oxygen. *J Am Dent Assoc.* July 2003;134.

Jackson DL, Johnson BS. Inhalation and enteral conscious sedation for the adult dental patient. *Dent Clin North Am.* 2002;46.

Jeske AH, Whitmire CW, et al. *Noninvasive assessment of diffusion hypoxia following administration of nitrous oxide-oxygen. Anesth Prog.* 2004;51(1).

Quarnstrum F, et al. Clinical study of diffusion hypoxia after nitrous oxide analgesia. *Anesth Prog.* January–February 1991;38(1).

Quarnstrom F. Nitrous oxide analgesia. What is a safe level of exposure for the dental staff? *Dent Today.* April 2002;21(4).

Malamed SF, Clark MS. Nitrous oxide-oxygen: a new look at a very old technique. *J Calif Dent Assoc.* May 2003;31(5).

Malamed SF. Sedation: *A Guide to Patient Management.* 4th ed. St. Louis, MI: Mosby; 2003.

Moore K, Dalley A. *Clinically Oriented Anatomy.* 4th ed. Philadelphia, PA: Lippincott, Williams & Wilkins; 1999.

National Institute for Occupational Safety and Health (NIOSH) Publication No. 96-107. NIOSH Technical Data Sheet, NIOSH Website: http://www.cdc.gov/niosh/nitoxide.html

Seifter J, Ratner A, Sloane D. *Concepts in Medical Physiology.* Philadelphia, PA: Lippincott, Williams & Wilkens; 2005.

Stedman's Medical Dictionary. 28th ed. Baltimore, MD: Lippincott, Williams & Wilkins; 2006.

Sweitzer B. *Handbook of Preoperative Assessment and Treatment.* Philadelphia, PA: Lippincott, Williams & Wilkins; 2000.

Wynbrandt J. *Excruciating History of Dentistry: Toothsome Tales & Oral Oddities from Babylon to Braces.* New York, St. Martin's Press; 1998.

Zacny J, Hurst B. et al. Preoperative dental anxiety and mood changes during nitrous oxide inhalation. *J Am Dent Assoc.* January 2002;133.

Zwemer TJ, et al. *Mosby's Dental Dictionary.* St. Louis, MI: Mosby; 2004.

Index

Page numbers followed by *f* or *t* indicate figures or tables, respectively.